Exploring BDSM:

A Workbook for Couples (or More) Discovering Kink

MORGAN THORNE

Exploring BDSM: A Workbook for Couples (or More) Discovering Kink
ISBN: 978-0-9958780-4-4

www.MsMorganThorne.com

Published by:
Nymphetamean Publishing
www.Nymphetamean.com
Toronto, Ontario

All content, including all text, photographs, and layout by Morgan Thorne.
Cover art & design by Morgan Thorne

Booksellers: For best results, display in the Sexuality section.

Warning & Disclaimer: This book is intended to be a reference guide and leaning aid. It is not a complete education on BDSM. The author strongly advises that people get in person instruction from an experienced instructor prior to engaging in BDSM activities.

The author and publisher assume no responsibilities for any injuries, loss, or damages resulting from the ideas presented in this book. The practice of BDSM comes with significant risks and while these can be lessened, they still exist. The use of drugs or alcohol greatly increases these risks. By acting on the information in this book, you assume all responsibility for your actions

Contents

1 EXPLORING BDSM: INTRODUCTION

Welcome to Exploring BDSM: A Workbook for Couples (or More!) Discovering Kink! Exploring the world of BDSM can be a little daunting for most people. This guide is intended to take you through the most common aspects of kink, step by step, and will allow you to try lots of different types of play.

Of course, if there is anything here that doesn't appeal to you, feel free to skip that section. Kink is meant to done your way - whatever works for the people involved is a-okay. The only universal is consent. We will get into the nitty-gritty of consent later, but it is the cornerstone of BDSM and it is what separates what it is we do (WIIWD) from abuse.

The first section of this book goes over the basics. We will talk about consent and negotiation, safe words and signals, aftercare, and typical mistakes that newbies make - and how to avoid them.

After that, we will explore different areas of BDSM play and D/s relationships. Each exploration follows the same pattern; you will fill out a BDSM checklist for each section, select a few activities that are highly ranked by both of you, try them out, and talk about what worked and what didn't a few days later. Each section also has safety information and other important things to know that pertain to that type of activity.

The checklists will also help you figure out what your specific hard and soft limits are. These are things that you don't want to do under any circumstances and things that you don't really want to do, but may try to make your partner happy.

The idea here is to show you a healthy, consensual, and safe way to explore your kinky fantasies with a partner (or more). Many people read fantasy or romance novels and try to recreate their favourite scenes, without understanding the basis of BDSM. Without the foundational skills and a basic understanding of how to approach play, those experiences can turn out badly. One partner may feel unintentionally violated or get accidentally hurt.

Exploring BDSM in a methodical manner may not seem as exciting on the surface - what with having to actually talk about your specific fantasies - but it is a much more rewarding experience in the end.

What is BDSM?

BDSM ends up having many different definitions, depending on who you talk to. The most basic is simply that it is an acronym for Bondage, Discipline, Domination, Sadism, Submission, and Masochism. Some people will say that the Domination and Submission (D/s) aren't part of the acronym - and they weren't in the very beginning - but they are an accepted part of it now.

Bondage is pretty straightforward. Anytime you bind a partner, using rope or leather cuffs, it falls under the bondage category. Things can get pretty creative and include items like pallet wrap for mummification or latex vacuum beds. Bondage is incredibly popular in kink culture, both as an element of a play scene or as a scene in and of itself. Shibari/kinbaku, Japanese style rope bondage, has become so popular over the last 10 years or so that it went from being a rare thing to a common sight at any party.

Discipline is doling out punishments for wrongdoing or breaking agreed-upon rules within a relationship. This is actually a somewhat rare practice in the world of BDSM. What is very popular is "Funishment" - role-playing punishments because it can be fun and sexy. Many people have eroticised the idea of being punished. It's not a good idea to break actual rules to try to get what you want and it's also a poor idea to reward bad behaviour. That's where the idea of funishment comes in. No rule breaking needed, you can make up a transgression or simply funish someone for having a 'smart mouth'. We will talk about the actual use of punishments briefly, but it's best to research in more detail if it's something you're interested in.

Domination is accepting authority within the bounds of a consensually negotiated power exchange relationship. A bit of a mouthful there? It's basically being in charge in the areas that you and your partner(s) agree on. A person can be a bedroom-only dominant or a 24-7 dominant who is always in control of the relationship and the submissive.

Submission is the flip side of Domination. Submissives give up authority within the bounds of a consensually negotiated power exchange relationship. They can be bedroom-only, or 24-7. They can have limits and boundaries (most do).

It should be obvious that D/s relationships take a lot of trust. Very few people start the relationship in 24-7 mode, so don't worry if that sounds daunting to you. There are plenty of people who enjoy bedroom-only D/s or power exchange that only happens for limited time frames (like a weekend). Remember, when it comes to kink, you do you!

Sadism, in the context of BDSM, is getting pleasure from causing consensual pain. This can be sexual pleasure or a different type of enjoyment. Pain can be physical, like a spanking, or emotional, like humiliation. It may sound a little odd, but remember, for every person that enjoys giving something, there is usually a person who likes receiving it.

Which brings us to masochism. Masochists, in the context of BDSM, enjoy being on the receiving end of sadism - they like pain. Again, they could get a sexual thrill from it or other forms of pleasure. There is a stereotype of the Dominatrix yelling "worthless worm!" at a submissive - while real life doesn't usually look like that, it does have a basis in reality. Some people really enjoy being humiliated, just like some people really enjoy a good beating.

The key to all of this, as I mentioned above, is that it is consensual. The people involved have talked about it and agreed to play with these ideas and activities. They have set up boundaries that feel comfortable to them and have a way to stop things if something goes wrong or it isn't as much fun as they think it will be.

When you begin exploring BDSM, you will need to talk about it. Negotiation is one of the most important skills a kinky person can learn. It can also be one of the hardest. So let's get into talking about our fantasies, negotiating reality and getting consent.

2 EXPLORING BDSM:

CONSENT IN BDSM

No matter how far into the world of BDSM you choose to explore, there will be one constant that you will hear: consent. Consent is what separates what we do from abuse. Consent is the foundation of BDSM. Consent is the line between kink and assault. Consent is...Well, you get the picture, consent is important!

What exactly is consent and how does it work within the framework of BDSM?

Consent Styles In BDSM

Consent is the voluntary agreement to participate in an activity. There is more to it, a lot of nuances, but that's it in a nutshell. Let's look at the different types of consent and then hammer out what our BDSM consent model should look like.

Implied Consent

Implied consent is the assumption of consent. You don't ask your romantic partner for consent every time you want to hold hands or kiss, you simply assume consent. This is partially because it's what is expected of romantic partners and also because you (presumably) obtained consent for those actions at some point in the past. Of course, if your partner pulled their hand away or turned their face when you tried those actions, you would understand that they have withdrawn their consent for those actions, and likely ask why. Depending on the reason, you may be hesitant and ask for consent the next time you wanted a kiss.

BDSM can make use of the implied consent model, but it's not the 'go to'. Most kinksters will want to obtain clear consent before an action or activity, often multiple times before moving to an implied consent model. This caution is for a good reason. Many of the things we do are dangerous, can be considered assault if done under the wrong circumstances, and receptiveness to an activity can very much depend on mood or prior agreements.

When you first start exploring BDSM, it is better to avoid the use of implied consent until you and your partner(s) find a comfortable rhythm - or have a conversation where you grant each other blanket consent.

Blanket Consent

Blanket Consent is where partners will grant permission for a specific activity or type of activity in all or most future encounters. It can be as simple as one partner saying "Anytime you want, you can grab me by the hair and kiss me - except in front of our families/kids". That permission would stand until it is specifically revoked, again either by stating it or when the relationship is dissolved.

Blanket consent can also cover more general activities. It is not uncommon for Dominants to ask for and be granted blanket consent for sexual activities with their submissives. They are allowed sexual access to the submissive whenever they want. Some couples will put restrictions on this access - only certain sexual acts, not during menses, not when the submissive is under a lot of pressure from work/school, etc. Others are granted total consent, even when the submissive isn't in the mood.

Of course, there are many other relationships where this type of blanket consent is not wanted or appropriate. If it's something you think you would enjoy, try it out. If it's something that makes you cringe, don't do it. There are Dominants and submissives of all sorts, compatibility is key here.

Affirmative Consent or Expressed Consent

Affirmative Consent or Expressed Consent is a consent model that relies on the clear expression of permission. This is where we will hear the saying "only YES means YES". It stresses that consent must be explicit and clearly given, and that anything other than a "yes" is a "no". Demurring means no. Avoiding means no. Nervous giggles mean no.

Consent in this model does not need to be verbal, although the verbal aspect is often the one that gets highlighted the most. A smile and a nod can be a yes. A thumbs up can be a yes. Since we are all kinky here, having your partner beg is a particularly fun way for them to say yes!

This form of consent can also be called enthusiastic consent. The idea between the two are very similar, however, there is one important difference. Enthusiasm isn't always needed for consent. You may not be enthusiastic about a dirty job while at work, but you still do it. In power exchange relationships, one partner may tell another to do something they don't really want to do, but the idea of obedience is important to both of them. They may consent to do the thing they're not into - sexual acts, chores, anything really - because it makes their partner happy and being obedient makes them happy.

This may sound like a strange or even unpleasant concept, but it is not uncommon in the BDSM world. I will stress again: if it's not for you, that's perfectly okay!

Consensual Non-Consent & Resistance Play

Consensual Non-Consent (CNC) is a relationship style in which the submissive/bottom/etc agrees to obey the dominant/top/etc, even when they don't really want to. They grant blanket consent to the top/dominant to do what they choose and are unable to withdraw consent.

This is not a very common relationship style within the world of BDSM. It is generally seen by people who practice 24/7 style relationships - a smaller portion of kinksters to begin with - and not all participate in CNC relationships.

CNC is a relationship style that takes immense amounts of trust and compatibility. It is not typical for a relationship to start as a CNC arrangement, rather it is something that develops over time as trust builds. People involved in these types of relationships try to find partners who have similar wants and limits to them so that they are not agreeing to do things that are disagreeable to them.

Some people in CNC relationships will negotiate limits, others enter into a "no limits" relationship. This sounds more extreme than it really is since compatibility has already been established. People with a clown phobia aren't usually going to engage in this style of relationship with someone whose clown fetish is of the highest importance to them.

It is important to understand the difference between CNC relationships and resistance play scenes.

Resistance Play is a scene where "no" doesn't mean stop. This is the type of scene where safe words are so important. If you have agreed that "no" or "stop" will be ignored, you need some way to communicate when things are wrong or if you need to withdraw consent.

Typical types of resistance play include ravishment (rape) play, kidnap scenes and any scene that plays with the idea of distress. I've even engaged in tickle scenes that were also resistance scenes - think about how you're going to struggle and yell when getting tickled relentlessly.

These two different concepts - resistance play and CNC relationships - have been conflated in recent years. Many older kinksters will correct and point out the difference but not everyone is aware. If you want to engage in either, it is imperative that you have a discussion about what exactly you are looking for.

Conditions of Consent

A yes doesn't mean very much if it's given by a person too drunk to understand what's going on or by a person who has no idea what they are getting themselves into. There are some conditions that absolutely need to be met in order to truly obtain consent.

Informed Consent

Informed Consent is consent given with an understanding of the typical risks and rewards of an activity. All parties involved must have knowledge of the potential consequences and be willing to take on any risks associated with the activity.

When you need surgery, the doctor will explain the procedure and detail the risks involved in having the surgery. They will also tell you what outcome you can expect and what to expect if you don't have the surgery.

BDSM is similar. There are risks to what we do. Sometimes those risks are small and easily mitigated. Other times, those risks are larger and harder to mitigate. Some activities take a high degree of skill to perform in a safer manner.

Understanding the risks as well as what you can expect to get out of a scene is important. Knowing what safety precautions are in place, the skill level or experience of your partner is also important.

It is generally expected that the top/dominant will be in a position to inform the bottom/submissive of the potential risks of an activity. There are times when this isn't the case, but they are the exception, not the rule. If you are a top or dominant, this is part of the responsibility that comes with the role.

Some Notes on Learning When You're New

An experienced and skilled bottom can help a new top navigate some complicated BDSM activities. A dominant who has attended classes to hone their skills can help guide an inexperienced bottom and keep them as safe as possible. Of course, partners who are new can also explore together, they just need to be even more vigilant regarding research and education. Learning together can be a lot of fun as long as everyone is open and honest about their skill level.

How do you know what you don't know when you're new? Do the research! Some bottoms think that because they won't be directing the action, they don't need to know anything about it. That can be true if you have a skilled partner you can trust. If not, you will need to know enough to tell a skilled person from someone blowing smoke. If you're into a certain activity, read about it, ask others in your community, take a class, do what you feel is right to learn enough to identify a safe partner.

New Tops/Dominants should spend a lot of time reading, talking to others, taking classes, observing, and taking in as much information as they can. Don't feel like you need to learn everything at once. Pick something and get good at it. Practice on inanimate objects as much as possible. Always be honest with your partner about your skill level. An experienced bottom can teach you as much as another top, so don't discount them as a valuable resource.

State of Mind & Consent

State of mind is important for giving consent. An intoxicated person can not give consent. Likewise, a person who is pressured or coerced cannot give consent. A person can not abuse a position of authority to obtain consent.

Coercion

As we talked about in the definition of consent, the agreement to participate must be voluntary. If a person is pressured in any way, then consent has not really been obtained. This can include social pressure or peer pressure, where a person feels they must comply because "everyone else is/does". It can be difficult in some situations to know when consent has been given freely and where some form of pressure has been expressed. If you have any doubts as to the authenticity of the consent given to you, it is much better to err on the side of caution and not proceed.

You should never be the one putting pressure on someone. If you are giving ultimatums or saying "if you loved me, you would...." the result is not consent. Coercion to get the answer you want to hear is not consent. Just like getting someone intoxicated because you think they are more likely to say yes is manipulative and does not result in consent.

Sadly, a common pressure tactic used often in the kink world is "you're not a real sub unless you..." or "I guess you're not a true dominant...". Both of these are manipulative tactics used to get one's way. If anyone says either of these things to you (or anything similar), your best bet is to walk away. These phrases are the mark of a person who does not respect your boundaries or consent.

Intoxication

Intoxication can be a tricky situation. What if you both sit down and have a few drinks, get a bit frisky and decide to have some fun. Is consent possible in this situation? Is either party responsible for the lack of consent? Does blame lie with the more sober person?

Even the law has a hard time answering these questions. Personally, I prefer to avoid any potential issues altogether and not play while intoxicated. If I or my partner(s) have had more than a drink or two, then BDSM play is not happening.

You will need to find your own comfort zone with this. How much can you imbibe before your judgment is impaired? Do you partake in other substances that can impair judgment? What about your partner(s)?

Some people choose to come to an agreement ahead of time regarding what can and can not happen if one or all parties are intoxicated. Some choose to remove more risky activities but say that simple things like spanking is okay. Others choose, like me, to abstain from play all together. You may also want to consider your local laws. Some (if not most) jurisdictions deem prior consent inadmissible at worst or rocky at best. This could land you in legal trouble, on top of the moral issues surrounding intoxication and consent.

Withdrawal of Consent

Consent can be withdrawn at any time before or during a scene. If the person you are with says no or uses a safe word (whatever you have in place to indicate that consent is no longer granted), and you continue - top or bottom, dominant or submissive - then you have violated that person's consent.

Consent can also be withdrawn for any reason. If a spanking is getting too intense for the participants, either one of them can withdraw consent. The top/dominant by stopping the activity and the bottom by saying stop or using a safe word (whichever they have agreed on). It is best to talk about why the scene or activity needed to stop - why was it too intense? Were the hits too hard? Was the bottom wanting more than the top was comfortable giving? Did the top go too hard too quick? Were there other elements, like humiliation, that either party weren't comfortable with?

Subspace & Re-Negotiating During Play

Subspace is an altered state of mind that bottoms/submissives can find themselves, in which they experience intense feelings of euphoria or other emotions. They can feel "floaty" or disconnected from their bodies. It is thought that subspace is caused by the endorphin rush that often accompanies play, but not everyone subscribes to this belief.

Some - no one really knows how many - bottoms and submissives experience this sort of altered state when playing. They may become non-verbal, they may feel more submissive or have strong urges to do everything they are told, and an intense desire to please.

top or dom Space is a similar state of mind, just the flip side of the coin. It is a mental state, often referred to in psychology as a "flow state" where everything feels like it's happening in perfect harmony. Athletes and artists often refer to this feeling as being in "the zone".

Since it is possible that both partners can enter into an altered state during the course of play, it is unethical to try to re-negotiate the scene in the middle. It can be frustrating if you think of the perfect thing to do part way through a scene, but you didn't negotiate it beforehand. I know, I've been there and done that. The best thing to do is make a mental note to talk about that activity later, use it in your next scene, or agree that it's okay to do on a whim. What you should not do is surprise your partner in the middle of the scene with something you haven't negotiated or discussed (unless you have a CNC style relationship).

Consent Culture

Within the world of BDSM, you will frequently see conversations about consent. These are important discussions to have - our understanding of consent is always evolving. The idea of asking for and getting consent is much more nuanced now than it was more than 20 years ago when I started in the kink world.

Kinksters are trying to create a consent culture, a place where consent is highly valued. The discussions may seem tedious to some, the rules may feel restrictive to some, but they are the best we have been able to come up with so far.

In BDSM, we never really stop learning. There are always more skills or new techniques. Your approach to consent should be the same - there is always more you can learn to ensure that your relationships and interactions are held to the highest standards of consent.

It is also important not to blame victims of consent violations, especially if you are the victim. Self-blame is tragic and common. Violators try to frame the situation so that they appear innocent and the victim appears to have done something wrong or is lacking in some way. It makes me sad that in this day and age - and in this community - that victim blaming still happens, but it does.

Do your best to support and encourage consent culture in your home, community, and relationships. Always ask for consent and respect a person's right to decline. Accept rejection with as much grace as you can. Support those who speak out against consent violations.

3 EXPLORING BDSM:

SAFEWORDS

Safewords can be strangely controversial in BDSM. You would think that any tool used for expression would be welcomed by people who emphasize the importance of communication.

The controversy comes from how common safe words are, how easily they can be misunderstood, and how rarely they are really needed. That may sound a little strange, so let me explain.

Safewords can mean different things to different people. In general, safewords are words that indicate that something is wrong or a withdrawal of consent. They can mean that partners should check in or stop the scene entirely.

That's part of the problem right there - what if you think "RED" means stop everything right away and I think it means to ask what's wrong, fix it, and continue on with the scene? That has the potential to be very damaging to the person who wants the scene to stop if they are the bottom. Both definitions are totally valid, so it's important to agree on what these words mean.

When you meet new people and decide to plan a scene, some will ask "what's your safe word?" as if everyone has one already. More and more I see people saying things like "if you don't have a safe word, you're not safe" and that it's a red flag for a dominant/top to not use a safe word.

For me, the only time a safe word is really needed is when you are engaging in some form of resistance play. At any other time, I take "no" to mean no and "stop" to mean stop.

Basically, unless we have taken the power away from those words, in a negotiated and consensual manner, I take what you say at face value.

Now, most dominant/tops I know will also heed any universal safe word. So even if we haven't agreed on a particular safe word, if you yell RED in the middle of a scene, I'm going to ask what's wrong and what needs to change. Heck, if you yell EGGPLANT in the middle of a scene, I'm going to at least check in!

You can see the problem here though. Misunderstandings can happen easily, especially when we are playing with dangerous themes like resistance. We play this way because it can be fun, but there is also a lot of risks involved.

Tops/dominants can use safe words too. They usually don't because they can simply stop the play if they need to, but there are some situations where they may need to use a safeword. For instance, if a top is "forcing" a bottom to perform oral sex, and the sensation is getting to be too much or not what they want, they could use a safe word to get the bottom to slow down or stop. They could also just issue an order, but if you're playing with a brat, that may backfire...(Again, any scene where you ignore plain language should be discussed ahead of time).

In the end, whether you use safe words or not is up to you and your partner(s). You can play the way I do, where words retain their meanings unless we agree otherwise. You can have a safe word in place for every single scene you do. You can use universal safe words or create your own. You can decide what those words mean for you or you can go with commonly accepted definitions. BDSM is what you make it, so have fun and do what works for you.

Universal Safe Words

I mentioned universal safe words above. What I mean by that are the words that are generally used as safe words in most dungeons, no matter where you are. These are words like RED and YELLOW as well as SAFE WORD. Pretty much wherever you are, people will recognize these as safe words and a need to stop play, at least temporarily.

Red often means stop the scene completely. I tend to shy away from this meaning of the word because I feel like it discourages bottoms/submissives from using it. What if they need me to stop the particular thing I'm doing, but don't want to end the scene? They may try to tolerate the thing for as long as possible, hoping that I will do something different.

If Red, or whatever safe word you choose, instead means "check in with me, something is wrong", the bottom/submissive is much more likely to use it. I can ask what is wrong, find out that the toy I'm using is unbearably painful but they wish to continue. I can then put that toy aside and continue the scene, knowing that both of us are enjoying it.

Of course, if red means check in, they can say they need to stop the whole scene at that point too. We haven't lost anything, but we have gained a way to correct problems without having to stop.

Yellow is often used to indicate that things are getting close to the limit for the bottom/submissive. The top/dominant can then use this information to push a bit further and end the scene, or back off and do something else to continue the scene. It gives the warning before red.

If we think of it in the same way as a traffic light, which can include green, then we can see how each colour works. These colours can also be used when we check in, by asking "what's your colour?". The answer we get can tell us a lot. Green can mean "Doing great! Keep up that intensity!" or "Good, keep going harder!" so you will want to decide on its definition.

The big advantage of these universal safe words is that if you are playing at a party or dungeon, other people will understand them as safe words. So if you are playing with someone who decides to disregard your repeated RED, you can be confident that someone else will step in to help.

Choosing a Safe Word

If you don't like the universal safe words, you don't have to use them. I generally encourage people to use the universal ones, just because they are universal. It's less to remember when distracted by the feelings of play.

Still, they won't work for some people. If you want to create your own safe word, keep these things in mind;

- Your safe word should be easy to remember. It does you no good if you need to use it and can't remember what it is.
- It should be easy to say. While using the name of a volcano in Iceland (Eyjafjallajökull, anyone?) may seem funny or clever, how on earth are you realistically going to use it?
- Shorter words are best, ideally only one syllable. This goes along with the ease of saying and remembering the word. Simple words are easiest to say and remember.
- It should not be a word that you (or another person) would reasonably say during a play scene. "Ouch" makes a terrible safe word, just ask any sadist! Your safe word should be something that is out of place in a BDSM scene, hence my eggplant example earlier. You wouldn't want your safe word to be confused with a request.
- You should have a discussion with every partner you have regarding the meaning of your specific safe word. You should also remind your partners before beginning that you use a different safe word, what it is and what it means to you. For those who play with multiple people, it can get a bit confusing and hard to remember without a regular reminder.

Safe Signals

Sometimes you just can't speak. Whether it's because you've had too many orgasms to form a coherent sentence or because your mouth is full with a gag, you do need a way to let your partner know something is wrong.

Safe Signals are a nonverbal cue that something is amiss. They could take the form of an object that makes noise, something that gets dropped or even a series of taps or grunts.

Common safe signals are a ball or keys that can be dropped. Keys will make noise, so many people prefer them. They are also something that most people will have on hand. A scarf can be used as a flag, to wave if you need to communicate something. The only problem with visual only signals is that they can be missed if your partner has their back turned.

Many people choose to "tap out" in the same way you would during a wrestling or MMA match. I like to use this signal myself. It does mean that I need to stay close to my bottom/submissive when they are gagged or unable to speak. If I am further away, they can tap on the furniture, but this can be hard to hear. This also means that I can't have them in really restrictive bondage, so I will sometimes use other safe signals, depending on the scene.

Some people will use grunts as a safe signal. For instance, three rapid, short grunts can mean check in. This is a great solution if you are restricting the ability to talk while using strict bondage where dropping an item or waving a flag would be difficult or impossible.

How to React to a Safe Word

How one reacts to a safe word can mean the difference between someone who violates consent and someone who respects it. It can mean the difference between an asshole and a good person.

Obviously, if you ignore a safe word and continue doing what you want, you will cross the line of consent. Remember that a safe word is used to indicate if something is wrong or to indicate a withdrawal of consent. If something is wrong, the person is going to withdraw their consent if you don't fix whatever is wrong. This should be obvious, but sadly, it needs to be said.

Furthermore, a person should never, ever, under any circumstances be ridiculed or punished for using their safe word.

I've seen some new Dominants, who maybe don't fully understand what purpose a safeword serves, saying that they punish a submissive if they use their safeword X amount of times. This is wrong on so many levels.

I understand that they think they know best when a safe word should be used. Dominants aren't mind-readers, how do they know if the submissive has a cramp, is going to throw up, or something is cutting off circulation?

Discouraging the use of safe words is encouraging unsafe play. Some bottoms/submissives will already not use a safe word when they should, for fear of causing disappointment (more on that in a bit). They should not be further discouraged.

If you are with someone who you feel is using their safe word frivolously, you really should have a talk with them. Find out why they are doing it and what could be changed to fix the situation. I have encountered some who think that using a safe word frivolously is fun or bratty behaviour. I try to impress on them the seriousness that most kinksters take safe words. It's not cute or bratty to call 911 because you're bored or want to get a rise out of someone. Using a safe word can be looked at in a similar way. It's there to be used if there is an emergency.

If I had a partner who insisted on playing around with the use of safewords, I wouldn't punish them. I just wouldn't play with them anymore. To me, that's a mark of an unsafe partner. How will I know when they are just playing around vs when there is a real emergency? It means I can't trust them and trust is so important to BDSM relationships.

I've also seen bottoms/submissives teased and ridiculed for using a safeword. People are competitive by nature, and bottoms/submissives are no different. Some view the ability to take pain or whatever their partner dishes out as a point of pride. Making fun of them for the use of a safeword can reinforce those competitive thoughts and cause them to ignore their own limits to the point they become injured. It can also add to any feelings of shame that they may have. Submissives/bottoms should not feel shame for using a safeword but some do, we don't want to make this situation worse.

Discomfort Around Safe Words

Not everyone is going to be comfortable using a safe word right off the bat. They may have had a previous partner who punished or ridiculed them for using one. They may be a competitive person who places great pride on being able to withstand more than others. They may not want to disappoint their partner. They may feel shy speaking up for their own needs. There are probably a hundred other reasons that someone may be hesitant to use a safeword.

It is important to always listen to safe words. No matter what. Even if you're having fun. Every single time one is used, you need to check in or stop (whatever is agreed on).

This will help reinforce the idea that the bottom/submissive is respected and cared for. They can see the evidence that we care more about their well being than our own fun.

Of course, reacting with concern is important. It defeats the purpose if you stop but get moody over it. Show your genuine concern. Do your best to rectify the situation. Really make sure you're putting your partner's needs in this situation above your own. This is one of the responsibilities that comes along with being a top/dominant.

If you have a partner who is reluctant to use their safeword, you can help them to normalize it. I will start to play with a gentle warm-up and have a quick reminder conversation at this time. I will ask, "What is your safe word?" and make them say the actual word. Next is, "What is your safe word used for?" and make them answer the question. Finally, I ask them to promise me they will use it when they need. I may, instead, tell them that I expect that they will use it under those circumstances and that I will be disappointed in them if they don't.

Which approach you use is up to you. I am assuming that you know your partner well enough to know which approach will work best. There may be other ways to reinforce the use of a safe word that suits your partner better, so feel free to improvise.

Finally, sometimes when playing, if things start to get really intense, you may be wondering if your bottom/submissive is still doing okay. You don't want to mess with their head space or the scene by flat out asking, so you can remind them that there is a way out while teasing them at the same time. Pick a noise they are making, whether it's "ouch" or just a grunt. Remind them that "Ouch is not a safe word!". This will hopefully remind them that there is a way they can stop things if they need to. I may also throw in "Calling me a bitch/asshole won't make me stop! That's not a safe word!".

This approach won't work for everyone, but it is a good way to remind your partner of your agreements without disrupting the flow of the scene. They may just be enjoying subspace so you don't want to disturb that if you can help it.

Of course, if there is ever any doubt in your mind that your partner is consenting, you need to stop and ask. Even if it ruins the flow of the scene. Even if it means you step out of "character" (if you are playing with personas or role play). I would much rather stop a scene because I was concerned about my partner than not stop and do them harm.

The more you play with someone, the better you will get to know them and their reactions. As you gain general BDSM experience, you will get better at reading body language. You will never become a mind reader though, so always err on the side of caution.

4 EXPLORING BDSM: NEGOTIATION

When you decide that you want to engage in BDSM, you can't just surprise your partner by grabbing them by the hair and spanking them. Well, you can, but it's really not a good idea. Without negotiation and consent, those actions become abusive, assault, and even sexual assault.

Negotiation is really just a fancy way of saying "talking about what you want to do and coming to an agreement". It's not, or shouldn't be, adversarial. It's not like a business negotiation, where the parties are each trying to get as much out of the other(s) as they can while giving up as little as possible. BDSM negotiation is much more friendly, sexy even. Each party (hopefully) wants to indulge the fantasies of the other in a way that they will also enjoy. It's about finding the common ground that you both (all) find exciting.

This is where the idea of BDSM checklists come in. BDSM Checklists are a list of possible activities that you fill out with a rating from "no way!" to "yes please!". They are a tool to help you find that common ground, that place where your kinks overlap. Filling out a checklist is helpful in the beginning, when you may not be sure what all the options even are. More experienced players will still use checklists for new partners because it can be an easy way to find out what the other is into. If it still seems a little odd, don't worry, we will be looking at checklists in more detail soon.

Once you know what you want to try, you need to talk to your partner about it. Checklists aren't consent. You still need to have the discussion and work out the details.

There are a number of things that you may want to consider when negotiating a scene. Some may be very important to you and others may not apply. The list later in the chapter is simply to give you an idea of what you may want to discuss.

Negotiations can also be different with different partners. If you are in a relationship that is sexually monogamous, but you have agreed to engage in BDSM play with outside people, you will negotiate differently with your romantic partner vs play partners.

Limits

Something that will come up in negotiations for BDSM play or D/s relationships are limits. There are two types of limits, hard and soft.

Hard limits are things you will not do under any circumstances. Most people will list the three "C's"; children, crap, and corpses. It's a little redundant since anything with children or corpses would fall into the category of crimes (a great fourth "C"), not kink, and crap (scat) is quite a rare fetish.

More realistically, people will list things that they are afraid of, blood and needles are a common limit in this category. Hard limits may also be things that creep them out, like clowns. It could be something that they have a visceral "NO WAY!" kind of reaction to, like impact play that leaves deep bruising. It can be things they've tried and found they really didn't like.

Your hard limits can be anything - and you don't have to explain your reasons to anyone unless you want to. If someone pressures or shames you about your hard limits, you may want to think about whether you really want to play with them.

Hard limits can also be things that you don't know how to do and don't have any desire to learn. It could be a thing that you don't feel comfortable doing to another person, for whatever reason. You will notice that these examples are coming from the top/dominant side of the slash because Tops/Dominants get to have limits too!

Soft Limits are things that you would rather not do but would consider doing for the right person or under the right circumstances. This could be things that you are nervous about and need someone that you really, really trust to guide you through it. It could be something you really don't enjoy, but your partner really loves, so you're willing to indulge them every once in awhile.

Just like hard limits, no one should shame you or give you a hard time about your soft limits. They also should not push those limits without your explicit consent.

And just like Tops/Dominants can have hard limits, they can have soft limits too. It could be things they are still learning and don't feel skilled enough to do to an actual person. It could be something that they share with their primary partner alone. It could be something that they will only do with certain people in private.

Whatever it is, everyone is entitled to have limits.

Pushing limits is the term that we use to describe play that pushes against pre-defined limits. So if clowns are a soft limit that you are willing to explore with your partner, big silly shoes or a red nose may be a way of pushing those limits without going full-blown clown.

Many kinksters believe that it is the person who holds the limit that should initiate the pushing. They should be the one who says "I think I might be ready to try this..." That way, there is no question of coercion. A person may feel pressured if their partner is asking about pushing one of their limits. If you are going to ask a partner to push a limit, a good rule is to ask once, then let them come to you.

Just as Tops/Dominants get to have limits and things that they don't feel comfortable doing, they may not feel comfortable pushing a partner's limits. They may feel much more comfortable playing with clearly defined consent and guidelines. This is okay! A person isn't any less of a top or dominant if they don't want to engage in pushing limits or if they don't feel comfortable pushing one specific limit.

Consent works both ways and everyone has to be in agreement before an activity can happen.

Negotiation Style

Negotiation isn't a one size fits all type of thing. There are many different approaches to negotiating a scene. Some styles are better suited to people you know well and are in an established relationship with, others are better for pick up play at a party.

Opt-In

Opt-in negotiation is probably the most simple approach to BDSM negotiations. You agree on which activities you want to do and that's what happens. No surprises, no random improvisation, just the specific things you have agreed to.

This style of negotiation works well in a few scenarios. First, it's great for pick up play or one-off scenes at parties. It's also great if you don't know your partner all that well, but still, want to play. You don't have to worry about figuring out if they will like this or that - it's all right there on the table.

I also like this style of negotiation when you are first starting to explore BDSM with a partner. Even if you've been married for 20 years, this is new territory for you. It's not the partner that's new and unknown, it's BDSM and your reactions to it. This is especially true if both (all) of you are new to kink. You may know what you've fantasized about, but reality can be a totally different beast.

Opt-Out

Opt-out negotiation is where you sit down and discuss what is off the table. This would be your hard limits and maybe your soft limits (depending on if you want to 'push' limits). Anything else is fine to do.

You can see why this style of negotiation is a bit more dangerous. It really should be reserved for people who know and trust one another deeply. You want to know your partner well enough to know what they are into and whether you are compatible with those things.

It's also a good idea to wait until you better understand what the world of BDSM entails. While it is unrealistic to expect any person to have a full understanding of everything that could be considered a kink - I'm still surprised by some kinks, even after more than 20 years - you should be familiar with the more typical things.

It would be bad form to use opt-out negotiation to justify doing something obscure that you know most people wouldn't be into. Of course, not everyone is totally ethical, so this sort of thing happens. Once again, it is important to know who you're playing with when using this style of negotiation.

Consensual Non-Consent

Consensual non-consent (CNC) is more accurately a relationship style, where the submissive partner agrees to obey the dominant partner - and the dominant partner can 'force' the issue if needed. It's a form of blanket consent, the submissive partner consents in the beginning to anything the dominant partner wants.

Obviously, this style takes even more trust than even opt-out consent. The two models can often be closely related since the dominant partner has a lot of power in these scenarios.

In CNC, the submissive partner may be allowed to have hard limits, but soft limits are considered fair game. This is a much more extreme version of opt-out negotiating and most often covers the whole relationship, not just a single play scene or play time in general.

If CNC sounds scary to you, don't worry. It's not that common in BDSM and is usually reserved for people who have a fair bit of experience in knowing what they like and what they don't.

If the idea of CNC sounds exciting to you, but only for a scene or limited amount of time, exploring resistance play may be for you. Resistance Play is where partners can play with the idea of force or non-consent in a negotiated and safer way. It's still a risky thing to do, and we will go into much more detail on resistance play in the chapter "Exploring Taboo & Edge Play " .

What Should We Negotiate?

What you should or need to negotiate is going to be different for each scene or each partner that you engage with. Negotiating a non-sexual scene with a casual play partner may hit on some things, while a sexual scene with a new partner is going to be a different negotiation than the same scene with your long-term marriage partner.

We will go through a list (what can I say? I like lists) of things that you may want to negotiate when doing a BDSM scene. It's up to you which elements you choose to use and which you don't. If something doesn't apply, don't worry about it. If something covers a part of your relationship that you're comfortable without negotiating, that's totally fine. This list covers as much as possible as if the parties involved don't know much about each other. I prefer to cover as many bases as I can and leave it to you to take what you want or need from it.

Scene Details

These details are the basics of the scene. The who, what, where, kind of things. You will want to decide on these factors first, then get into the finer points of your scene.

Who will be involved in your scene? No one should ever join in on a scene without prior permission and consent of all the participants. "Surprising" your spouse with a third person is a terrible idea, even if you have talked about it in terms of fantasy before. If you are interested in adding more people to your mix, that will be discussed in detail in "Exploring Sexuality &Sexual Taboo" (page 154).

What 'feeling' do you want your scene to have? What do you want to get out of the scene? Do you have specific goals for this scene? If so, what are they and how can they be achieved?

Some of those questions may seem a bit odd. Morgan, you may say, we just want to have a bit of sexy fun! What's with the strange questions?

Well, a scene where you want it to be light-hearted and fun is different from a scene where you want it to feel dark and ominous. One feeling is great for an interrogation role-play scene, while the other may be better suited for a tease and denial scene.

Sometimes we may not know immediately what we want to do, but we do know how we want to feel. It can be a useful starting point for some people. If it doesn't work for you, skip it.

If you don't already have defined roles, who will take which one? Will there be switching mid-scene? Is this a scene where one person will have control or power? Is it a scene where one person will be performing actions without any specific power exchange?

If you are going to switch roles part way through, when does this happen? Is it a fight for control? Is it taking turns doing an action without power exchange? What will the switching look like?

Where will your scene take place? What are the restrictions on the place? Do you need to bring anything special into the space, or is everything you need already there? Who will bring what, if needed?

If you're playing at home, what do you need to take into account? Do you need to wait until the kids are in bed, then make sure you're quiet enough not to wake them? If that's the case, maybe a gag would be a good idea and you might want to avoid toys that make a lot of noise (or make the receptive partner make a lot of noise!). How can you work around those restrictions or make them part of play? Can you command your partner to be silent, then do that thing you know they love with the vibrator - it can be fun to watch them squirm and you can easily take away the vibrator as 'punishment' for disobeying.

If you're playing at a public dungeon party, what are the rules? If you prefer sexual scenes and they don't allow nudity or sex, how will you handle it? You could wait until the end of the night to do your scene after you're done socializing, so that you can go right home and hop into bed. If you're doing some sort of edge play (play that is generally considered to be more dangerous), do you need to bring anything special, like a sharps bin? Do you need prior permission from the party host or DM?

If you're playing at a hotel or a rented space, what do you need to consider? Are the walls thin so the neighbours can hear everything? If so, it may not be the time to do a resistance play scene. A visit from the police is not a good way to end a scene.

Are you playing in another space that needs special consideration? Outdoors is a popular fantasy for many people, but what are the chances and consequences of getting caught? Do you have some private land where you will be undisturbed? A public park may up the danger, but it's generally considered bad form to expose others to your kink - and could be illegal in the case of sexual play being exposed.

There are many places to play, but you do need to make sure that you have your bases covered. You are looking to have fun, not spend the night in jail!

Play may not always take place right after negotiation. Often, we will negotiate scenes a few days in advance, especially if playing at a party. This can also be useful if you want to do some surprise play - you know what will happen, but not when.

I knew a couple who would negotiate 'kidnap' type scenes for parties. They worked out the details in advance, both went to the same party. She had a signal, like removing glasses, to show him when she was ready to play. Any time after that, he would grab her and the scene would begin. She never really knew when it would be - which was part of the fun.

How long will your scene last? Is it an evening? Until you're both tired and go to sleep? Until everyone has an orgasm? The weekend? You get the idea.

Knowing how long a scene is supposed to last can help avoid misunderstandings and hurt feelings. Most importantly, it can help avoid consent violations. If you're doing resistance play and one partner thinks the scene is over while the other thinks it's still going and ignores the word "no", there is a problem.

So you can see that even these seemingly small details can be very important to discuss. It may not take that long, but it's good to cover. In the beginning, negotiating will probably take a lot longer because you will want to check each item. As you grow more comfortable with it, you will know what applies and what doesn't, or what needs to be discussed and what doesn't.

Limits & Safe Words

Depending on what style of negotiation you've used, you may not need to go into explicit details regarding your hard and soft limits. It's wise to mention your limits so that your partner doesn't accidentally do something they shouldn't. For instance, if one of your limits is no hands on your neck/throat, and you've agreed to some rough play, some people might think that a hand on the throat is included in that. It's always best to err on the side of caution when it comes to limits and consent.

- If you are using safe words for your scene, what are they?
- Will you use the "universal" safe words of "red", "yellow", or "green"? Will "safe word", another universal safe word, be used?
- Will you use your own, personal safe word?
  - Is it easy to remember, for everyone involved in your scene?
  - Is it simple to say, even under stress?
- What is the meaning of your safe word(s)?
  - Do they mean stop or check in?
- Under what circumstances will you be using safe words?
  - To indicate a potential problem, like a leg cramp or too tight rope?
  - To indicate a withdrawal of consent?
  - To indicate a change of pace or other alterations in the scene progression?
- Will you be engaging in resistance play?

It is important to negotiate resistance play. If the top/dominant is not expecting resistance and the bottom/submissive starts yelling "no, stop!" it can be confusing and will probably stop the scene short. Unexpected physical resistance can end a scene with an angry top/dominant who deems the bottom/submissive an unsafe player. Clear communication in this area is essential to a good scene and maintaining a good relationship.

What are your hard limits for this scene or this partner? Will you be pushing limits? What does that look like to you? Pushing limits will be discussed in more detail in Exploring Taboo & Edge Play.

Are there any warning signs of a bad emotional state that everyone should be aware of? Under what circumstances should the scene stop if things aren't going well and the bottom/submissive isn't able to articulate a safeword?

Sobriety

Sobriety is generally expected among kinksters. Some people may feel comfortable doing more "mild" scenes, such as bare handed spanking, after having a few drinks or indulging in other mind-altering substances. Very few kinksters will feel comfortable playing when participants are drunk or high, although there are exceptions. Generally, BDSM is considered to be somewhat dangerous, even the "mild" stuff, so one should have their wits about them.

Occasionally, some people may want to include drunkenness or being high in a scene deliberately. This should be thoroughly negotiated beforehand between those involved and is considered edge play. If sobriety is not expected, what level of intoxication is acceptable?

Sexual Activity

What is sexual activity? What does it include? This list is going to be different for just about everyone. Most will agree that fondling genitals or intercourse is sexual activity, but what about massage, a caress, a kiss, or even sticking fingers in the mouth of another?

Sadly, there are many stories about people's consent being violated by partners who had a different understanding (or claimed to have a different understanding) of what constitutes sexual activity. While it won't stop bad people, it may let them know that you are savvy enough to negotiate thoroughly - allowing you to dodge the bullet of playing with them. It will also help avoid the genuine accidental violation due to miscommunication.

Now, you may not need to go into this much detail if you have a long-term established partner. In that case, you know what the other likes and what they don't like. Unless you're trying something new, all you have to agree on is if things will get sexual or not.

- Will this scene include sexual contact?
    - Sexual talk
    - Kissing
    - Nipple stimulation
    - Genital caressing/stimulation
    - Anal stimulation
    - Digital penetration (anus or vagina)
    - Oral sex?
    - Anal sex?
    - PIV?
    - Mutual masturbation?
    - Other activity
- Are the rules the same for everyone involved?
- If sexual contact is involved, what types of barriers or other precautions should be used?
    - Gloves?
    - Female birth control?
    - Pill, IUD, implant, ring, etc.
    - Dental dams?
    - External condoms (the common condom)?
    - Internal condoms (also known as female condoms)?
    - Spermicide?
    - Plastic wrap?
    - Barriers (condoms, etc) on toys?

Play Details

Here is where you will want to discuss the details of the play you want to do in the scene. For some, this will be the main part of the negotiation. For instance, if you have an established partner, you may not need to discuss other aspects of the scene in minute detail, you just need to agree on what kind of kinky fun you're going to get up to. For others, talking about each of these points will be important.

When you're new or new to each other, it's best to cover everything rather than miss something important. I promise it's not as boring as it may seem!

- What type of scene or what kinds of play will you be doing?
    - Impact?
    - Bondage?
    - Mind-fuck?

  - Humiliation?
  - Sensation?
  - Others
- Are marks permitted?
  - No marks
  - Lots of marks
  - Marks only where they can be easily hidden
  - Marks only on certain parts of the body
  - Temporary marks (few days - few weeks)
- Will you be engaging in degradation or humiliation?
  - Verbal humiliation?
  - Physical humiliation?
  - Public or private?
- Are there any words or actions that are off limits?
- What should be done in case of an emotional land-mine?
- What are your limits for this scene?
- What style of scene do you want to do?
  - Lots of laughter?
  - Light & fun?
  - Serious?
  - High protocol?
  - Bratty or talking back?
  - Crying?
  - Funishment?
- What are your favourite things that fall within the activities negotiated?
- What could be used as a reward, if applicable?
  - Favourite toy
  - Favourite type of play
- What do you really want to happen?
- What do you want to get out of the scene?
  - Orgasm
  - Catharsis
  - Fun
- Do you require aftercare?
  - What type?
  - Does your scene partner need to provide it, or is a surrogate okay?
- Do you experience drop?
- Do you need a check in the next day or a few days later?

Health Concerns

It is important to disclose any relevant health concerns to your scene partner before you begin. This is important if there is a medical emergency during or after the scene. It is also important so that your partner understands your limitations - a top/dominant with a bad shoulder isn't going to be able to throw a flogger for an hour straight, and a bottom/submissive with arthritis in their knees won't be able to crawl around on hard floors for any length of time. Talking about it ahead of time avoids awkward situations during the scene and helps to protect the health and well being of all involved.

This isn't limited to just physical health, mental health is important too. If there are activities that may trigger your depression or anxiety, you probably want to avoid those.

If you are unsure about whether a health condition is relevant, you may want to err on the side of caution. It is, of course, up to you - health information is very personal and it's understandable to want to keep some things to yourself.

If you have a condition that you fear may cause people to not want to play with you, it really is best to disclose. Many people rightfully fear stigma associated with some STIs. Many people in the kink community are fairly well informed about various STIs and will take a more measured approach. Like any group of people, there are those who will react badly - and you won't know until you disclose. I wish everyone was compassionate and understanding (even if they don't want to play with someone that has an STI), but that's not reality. More and more people are learning how to handle various STIs, so the stigma is slowly easing.

There are other health issues that can interfere with play too. A few years back, there was a story of a bottom who didn't disclose their seizure disorder to a top before they engaged in some pretty strenuous play. The top was understandably upset and angry. I had a person fail to disclose their Hepatitis C status before play that involved blood. I was unhappy at the lie by omission, but I always play as if all blood contains pathogens, so I wasn't worried about my health being affected.

You can see the importance, then, of disclosing your health status in many situations. It can help protect everyone involved. You may need to do some educating, on what to do in an emergency or how to handle things if something goes wrong. It's much better to have it all out in the open, rather than try to explain in the middle of a bad situation.

- Do you have any health issues that could affect the scene?
- Is there anything that should be avoided?
- What should be done in an emergency?
- Who to call?
- What is an emergency?

- At what point should you go to a hospital or call 911 (specific to your condition)?
- Do you have any medications that you may need in an emergency?
- What should your partner do with these if they are needed?
- Where can they be found? Is it easily accessible when you're stressed?
- Are there specific instructions on how to administer, if needed?

Relationships

For those who are playing casually, the question of what sort of relationships or obligations the partners have towards each other can be an awkward conversation to have. Even more awkward and potentially hurtful is not talking about it. I've encountered bottoms/submissives who felt that what I regarded as casual pick up play meant that we were in some sort of relationship. I've had others that I thought were more serious than they were, after many, many play scenes.

If you're playing within an established relationship, you may still want to check in to see if play changes how you normally relate. You may have a scene where you talk about the fantasy of a third person. If one of you takes that to mean it's okay to actually invite a third person to join you in bed, while the other thinks it's just fantasy talk...Well, you see where this is going!

- What sort of relationship are you in (if any)?
  - Play partners
  - Casual play
  - Romantic
  - D/s relationship
  - Monogamous
  - Polyamorous, open, swing, etc
- Does this play change any of your already established relationship rules or norms?
  - Are you now open to multiple partners?
  - Will you be transitioning to 24/7 D/s?

There are likely many more points that you could negotiate before a scene, depending on what you're doing and who you're doing it with. These are the basic points I like to hit before playing - of course, not every scene requires all of these questions answered. Use your discretion and do what works for you and your partner(s).

Negotiation can seem daunting in the beginning, with all these things to remember and your nervousness at even talking about kink. The important thing to remember is that it gets easier with time. You will get more and more used to talking about your desires and one day you will find yourself openly sharing your most perverted thoughts with relative strangers at a munch (or not, but that's how it worked for me).

You will also get used to the questions that you find important, which will become your personal negotiating style. You may find that some of the items in my list are unimportant to you, while I've maybe left out something you find essential. Change things up as much as you need.

Remember, it gets easier with time and practice, like pretty much anything. Muddle through the first few times and you will gain confidence. Negotiation is how you get your fantasies fulfilled - no one is a mind reader, we need to communicate our needs to each other.

5 EXPLORING BDSM:

ROLES IN BDSM

There are more roles in kink-land than you can shake a stick at, so for the purpose of this book (and so you don't end up hopelessly confused), we will take a look at some of the basic roles. If you find that none of these roles really does it for you, or you find a different role that speaks to you, use it.

These are a starting point. The roles I will be discussing here are more universal, they are most likely to be recognized by kinksters around the world. Some of the more specialized roles, like princess, are more individual and less common. Others, like kijara, are used within certain subsets of the BDSM community (in this case, Gor). Still others, like bull, are kink specific. I won't be going into detail on these types of roles (although some will get a quick explanation when we discuss kinks). If any of those appeals to you, feel free to look them up.

Role names can also vary depending on what community you are a part of. If you're gay and enjoy playing both top and bottom, you would be called versatile. Straight folks who enjoy the same thing are commonly known as switches. Whenever possible, I will try to provide these 'alternatives' and an explanation.

Finally, a quick note on roles. No one expects that a single word is going to sum up all that you are. Many people will use multiple roles to describe themselves. If it feels more comfortable for you to use multiple terms, go for it! Many of us pick one "umbrella" role that we most strongly identify with, then if the need to elaborate comes up, we will be more specific.

For instance, I generally identify as a Dominant. If asked for a single word to describe what I do in kink, that's it. If I need to elaborate, I can say that I'm also a top, a sadist, a lifestyle & professional domme, a master to my slave - and there are probably a few more that would describe me that I'm not thinking of right now.

Most importantly, if you are getting into a relationship of any sort with a person, you should explain what these roles mean to you. Definitions can be funny things, changing from person to person.

General Roles

These roles are more general and work as umbrella terms. A person may choose one of these identities if they are unsure about where they fall in the kink world, or if they feel the term resonates with them.

Vanilla

Vanilla may seem like an odd one to start with on a list of BDSM & kink roles, but many of us once identified this way - even if we didn't realize it. Vanilla is someone who isn't kinky, who has no interest in BDSM or D/s relationships. It should not be used in a derogatory sense, there is nothing wrong with not being kinky, just like there is nothing more 'advanced' about us because we enjoy some kinky sex or power exchange relationships.

Kinkster

A Kinkster is a person who has kinks, who participates in the kink community, or who engages in BDSM practices on their own. Often it's all three. Normally, people use it as a term that covers everyone who is involved in BDSM, D/s, or kink. Alternately, a person may identify as a kinkster if their interests in BDSM span a wide range of other identities.

Hedonist

While not a specific BDSM role, a Hedonist is a person who enjoys pleasure for pleasure's sake. The pursuit of pleasure is an overriding philosophy in their life, they focus on doing things which brings them (usually sexual) pleasure.

Fetishist

A Fetishist is someone who has interest in one or more sexual fetishes. In common use today, it can refer to people who are into BDSM in general, but the use is misguided (partially because of Fetlife, a popular BDSM website, conflates kinks with fetishes). A fetish is a sexual attraction to things which are not usually considered sexual, for example, foot fetishes. On the other hand, a kink is simply a BDSM activity, which may or may not include fetishes.

Mentor

A Mentor is a person who helps to teach someone, who acts as a wiser, more experienced advisor, and who can give advice to a person who is learning within the world of BDSM. Much like in the vanilla world, a mentor is someone who has experience that you lack and want to learn.

It is generally suggested that a mentor should be the same gender and kink role as you so that they can relate to your experience. The emphasis on kink role is greater than the emphasis on gender - a Dominant can learn a lot from another Dominant, no matter what gender either of them are.

Many people don't like the idea of Mentors, preferring to learn from many people or to attend classes on specific subjects. A person should not look for a mentor until they know what they want to learn. Again, like in the vanilla world Mentors are usually more experienced people you've formed a friendship with who share their knowledge freely.

Sexual relationships between Mentors and mentees are frowned upon. There has been a trend in the kink world (mostly online) recently where people use the term Mentor to manipulate people into a sexual relationship.

Mentors are falling out of favour now that there are so many different resources for learning in the kink community. Most people prefer to read books, watch videos, read blogs, take classes, and attend community events to learn new skills.

Power Exchange Roles

These roles are specific to power exchange relationships and have little to do with play or BDSM activities.

Dominant

A Dominant is a person who enjoys taking control of a consensually negotiated power exchange relationship. They have the authority to make decisions in the areas agreed to by both them and their partner(s).

Dominant has nothing to do with play activities, nor does it indicate a person's role when (and if) they engage in BDSM, such as spanking, flogging or bondage. A person can be a Dominant without doing any kinky activities, they are simply the leader in their relationship. This can be seen in Taken in Hand (an often Christian themed power exchange which believes that the man is the head of household).

There are as many styles of Dominant as there are Dominants. Most Dominants are not walking around barking orders to anyone and everyone (and those that do are set straight or kicked out of kink spaces rather quickly). Dominant is not synonymous with asshole or bitch.

Dominant is often capitalized. A quick way of expressing who is in charge of a relationship is to write the gender of the Dominant in a capital, followed by a slash, then the gender of the submissive. For example, a dominant woman and submissive man would be expressed as F/m. A dominant man with a submissive man would be M/m.

Variations on Dominant include;

- Dom - a gender-neutral shortening of the word Dominant. Many people take it to indicate a male person, but it can refer to any gender.
- Domme - a faux French word that indicates the Dominant is a woman. It came about during the early days of internet chat rooms and message boards. Pronounced in the same way as "Dom".
- Dominatrix - almost always indicates a professional, female dominant.
- Domina/Dominus - Latin for master or owner. The ending indicates gender; "a" is a woman and "us" is a man.
- Daddy or Mommy Dom - A person who has a nurturing or parental style of dominance. Can also be kink specific (see Mommy & Daddy in kink specific roles)
- Sir/Ma'am - an honorific used when speaking to a Dominant partner, but also used in reference to that partner, ie "My Sir said I was good".

Master

The term Master is a gender-neutral term used to indicate a person who is involved in a 24/7, usually total power exchange relationship. Can also indicate a person who consensually "owns" another person (again, in a consensually negotiated power exchange relationship).

Some people use Master to indicate a man or a masculine woman who fills this role.

Master can also refer to a person who is extremely skilled in an activity, or it can be a title bestowed by a community (see Leather).

Some people find it a hot term to use during play, which is why it's important to discuss what terms mean to you.

Variations on Master include;

- Mistress - indicates that the Master is a woman.
- Owner - a person who owns a slave or person
- Sir/Ma'am - used in the same way as with a Dominant. An honorific used to address the Master but also to refer to them.

SUBMISSIVE

Submissive is the complementary role for dominant. A submissive is a person who gives up control over things which have been consensually negotiated in a power exchange relationship. They agree to cede to the authority of their dominant.

Submissive has nothing to do with play activities, in the same way, that dominant does not. A person can be a submissive without engaging in any BDSM activities, or while engaging as a top for BDSM. Many submissives take on the role of bottom as well, but it is not universal and should not be assumed.

Much like dominant does not mean jerk, submissive does not mean weak. Submissive people are just as strong, independent, and confident as the rest of us (of course, they may not be confident, or they may be shy, or any number of normal human traits). While some people may enjoy humiliation as a kink, the things said during playtime should not be considered to be how the participants really feel. I mean, if a dominant really thought that a submissive was a "worthless worm" and the submissive also believed this, why would they be in a relationship together?

Variations on submissive include;

- Sub - a shortened version of the word submissive.
- Fem-sub - indicating a female submissive.
- Male-sub - indicating a male submissive.
- Subbie - an affectionate term for submissive. Be careful using it, unless you know the person you are referring to is okay with the term, some people find it offensive and derogatory to their role.
- Service Submissive - a submissive who gets fulfillment through being of service to others, whether to the community or to their specific dominant.
- House Submissive - a submissive who is in service to the "house", often a person in a service role at a high protocol party or similar events. They usually have well-defined roles (serving drinks, for example) and are not available for casual play by others at the party.
- Alpha Submissive - in a multi-submissive household or relationship, the submissive who holds the highest rank (if a ranking system is in place). They can act as a majordomo, delegating tasks to the other submissives and ensuring that the Dominant's will is carried out properly.
  Also a misused term to indicate that a person (usually male) is submissive but still "manly", "strong", or otherwise not a "worthless worm" type submissive (ignoring that manly, strong, etc. are common traits among male submissives and that submissives aren't weak, pathetic, or otherwise worthless in any way).
- Warrior Princess Submissive - A term used in the same way that alpha-sub often is. Originally coined by Michael Makai, a disgraced BDSM author who was charged and convicted of various sex crimes, including those that involved a minor. The term has

gained popularity among female submissives for the same reason that men use the alpha-sub title - a profound misunderstanding of what a submissive is.

Slave

Slave is the complement to master. A slave is a person who has agreed to give up all authority to their Master, usually in a 24/7 TPE style relationship. The extent of the power exchange will depend on what has been negotiated by the people involved and what they consent to.

Slave is gender neutral and is one of the few terms where there is generally no gender assumptions made about the person.

Some people may find it a term that is exciting to use during a play scene, so make sure you are on the same page as the person you are talking to.

Some people find the term slave to be offensive, considering the all too recent history in the United States of chattel slavery. This can be a source of controversy within the kink community, especially in parts of the U.S.

Variations on slave include;

- Property - a slave may be considered or prefer the term property. Often goes with the role owner.

Switch

A Switch is a person who can alternate between roles. In the case of power exchange roles, a person would identify with both the Dominant side and the submissive side. They may switch these roles with different people or at certain times with the same person. Switching D/s roles with the same person is more rare than switching Top/bottom roles with the same person.

Switch used in this way is common in both the gay and pan-sexual kink scenes.

Play Oriented Roles

These roles are the ones people take on during BDSM play. They often describe who is doing the action and who is receiving.

Top

A top is a person who performs an action. This could indicate the person who is giving the spanking, the person who is tying the rope, or the person who is using humiliating words towards another (depending on the type of scene). Topping does not always mean pain, a top may choose to give sensual pleasure, do sensation play, or any number of things that we will learn about later on. These actions are consensual and negotiated ahead of time.

Often, top and dominant go together in the same person, but not always. Some dominants like to bottom for certain activities, where they will command their submissives to top them. Some people are not interested in power exchange at all and just want to do kinky things. If they are performing the action, without any power exchange, they are the top.

Variations on top include;

- Service top - a person who tops (performs actions) as a service to another. Often, but not always, a submissive person.

Sadist

A sadist is a more specific version of top. A sadist is a person who enjoys giving consensual pain to another person. They may enjoy physical acts like spanking, or emotional acts like humiliation. In either case, these actions are negotiated ahead of time and are consensual in nature.

Variations on Sadist include;

- Sensual Sadist - a person who enjoys causing pain while also indulging in sensual or outright sexual play.

Bottom

A bottom is a person who is on the receiving end of actions performed by the top. They are the person getting the spanking, being tied up, or having humiliating things said to/about them. Bottoms are not always interested in pain, they may prefer to bottom for sensual or sensation type activities, or they may enjoy other types of play that we will discuss later on. These actions are consensual and negotiated ahead of time.

Bottoms are not always submissive, although there is a big correlation between the two. Many submissives also bottom, but some dominants enjoy bottoming as well. Other people enjoy bottoming without any power exchange at all.

Variations on bottom include;

- Power bottom - a bit of a controversial term, most agree that power bottoms are people who can take a lot of BDSM play, usually pain play. This comes from the gay usage of the term, a guy who can be on the receiving end of sex and last for a long time.
    - Some people will use the term to describe a dominant bottom, but this is not common.
- Sufferer/Sufferist - a person who is not masochistic but is willing to endure pain play and other discomforts to please or entertain the top or dominant.

Masochist

A Masochist ideally partners up with a sadist, each being one side of the same coin. Masochists are people who get pleasure from pain. They enjoy it in some way, sexual, non-sexual pleasure, a sense of pride, or even cathartic release. Some masochists can achieve orgasm from pain (referred to as a paingasm).

Masochists may be very specific about the type of pain they enjoy, while others enjoy any type of pain. Emotional masochists enjoy emotional pain, like humiliation. Masochist is usually assumed to mean the enjoyment of physical pain unless indicated otherwise.

Variations on masochist include;

- SAMs (Smart Ass Masochists) - these are people who like to mouth off to egg on the sadist or top, encouraging them to push harder and deliver more pain. This exchange is often playful in nature, and some do not enjoy engaging in this way.

Versatile / Switch

A person who is versatile or a top/bottom switch can alternate between the two roles. They enjoy the experience of topping as well as the sensations of bottoming. They may switch roles with the same person or prefer different roles with different people. Both are common with top/bottom switching.

Switch is used for both Dominant and submissive switching as well as top and bottom switching within the pan-sexual BDSM community. Versatile is used to denote top/bottom switching within the gay community (although it is being used more often in the pan-sexual community now).

It should also be noted that a person can switch both D/s and play roles, either with the same person or with different people.

Community Specific Roles

These roles are specific to various communities or subcultures within BDSM. Some may not identify as being kinky, but rather as having interest in power exchange relationships. When those objections or restrictions apply, I will make a note of it.

Leather

Leather began in the late 1940's and early 1950's with the rise of gay motorcycle clubs. Since then it has evolved into having multiple meanings, depending on who you talk to.

The first is that within LGBTQIA communities, leather means the same thing as kink or BDSM. A person who is kinky is into leather. This centred around the idea of leather bars, where kinky queers hung out and the dress code required a certain amount of leather (or other kink gear like latex) to get through the door. Many of these clubs did not cater to exclusively gay clientele either. Leather bars were once one of the few places that straight people could be openly kinky and it was a convenient way to seek out partners.

My first involvement with the kink community was through leather bars. As an asexual, I am firmly in the 'queer' camp, but I do date people of all genders, so leather bars were a natural fit for me.

The idea of a Leather Community came about when people who were into leather decided to adopt more formal, protocol-driven groups that held the values of brother/sisterhood, loyalty, duty to the community, and honour in high regard. This idea appealed to both queer and straight folk, and there are Leather groups to be found in both communities.

Leather is also where we get a lot of our ideas about how kink is done. The idea of starting out as a bottom and "working your way up" to being a top was started in some leather communities (not all of them use this model). Mentoring of novices, an experienced top/dominant taking a novice top/dominant under their wing (same with bottom/submissives), also began in with some leather communities who preferred this style of learning. The idea that there is a titular Master, something bestowed by the community, comes from Leather culture too.

The history of leather (or Leather) is fascinating and I can not do it justice in this space. If it is something that interests you, I encourage you to seek out your local leather group (most major cities have them) and learn.

Some terms associated with leather include;

- Leatherman - A man who is into leather (kink) or part of the Leather Community
- Leatherwoman (Leatherdyke) - A woman who is into leather (kink) or into the Leather Community. Leatherdyke is specific to lesbians.
- Old Guard - an overly romanticized idea that there was some perfect ideal of kink, specifically Leather, a community that was united in values, protocols, and respect for the universal rules of BDSM. This time never existed, the community as a whole has never had a set of universal rules, and there have always been people who are not into any sort of formal protocol.

  Now, when people call themselves Old Guard, they often practice this idealized version of kink as a personal style or it's because they have little to no real life experience in kinky communities.

Gor / Gorean

A high protocol version of BDSM, highlighting power exchange, that was created based on the books by John Norman. The Gor series are science fiction books which take place on an alternate Earth-type planet, called Gor. There is a strict patriarchal system in place, where women are literally slaves. Goreans, people who follow the philosophy laid out in the books, will often use language specific to the subculture.

Many try to distance themselves from kink and the BDSM community in general, claiming that they do not practice BDSM. Power exchange relationships are the focus of Goreans, with less emphasis on kink elements. When they do appear, it is usually in the form of genuine punishment.

I have done my best to provide accurate information about the Gorean way of life here, as short as this section is. I do not participate in this community, so there are going to be nuances that I miss. If you're interested in the idea of Gor, the first step is to read the novels. Then reach out online and you will find lots of others who enjoy the lifestyle as well.

One of the more famous elements of the books are the slave positions. These are various poses that serve practical and aesthetic purposes that Gorean slaves must learn. They have since been incorporated into many people's kink lives, some who have never even heard of Gor.

Terms associated with Gorean culture include;

- Kijara - a female, multi-purpose slave. She must be able to perform basic household tasks, such as cooking and cleaning, as well as being available for sexual use by her Master. There are also more specifically trained pleasure and passion slaves, who specialize in carnal delights.
- Kijarus - a male, multi-purpose slave. From what I understand, they are much less common than kijara.
- Free Woman - a woman who is not enslaved and can provide companionship to a male Gorean. In the books, only a free woman can bear children who are not slaves themselves. For those who are Goreans, the kijara can be freed temporarily in order to bear free children (since it's unethical to involve children in our kinks).

Taken in Hand

Taken in Hand relationships are male-lead power exchange relationships. Many will adamantly argue that they are not part of the umbrella of BDSM. Of course, a lot of them talk about ravishment (rape) play, discipline in the form of spankings, and other kinky activities. Some will identify as submissive or feel submissive to their husbands, but kink terminology is rarely used.

They are less familiar with the concept of consent than most kinksters, with many sites saying that if a wife doesn't seem unhappy or strenuously object, then the husband has consent to make unilateral decisions. Many accounts I have read seem to expect that the wife will not consent, and give advice on how husbands should enforce their will, regardless.

Some who participate in Taken in Hand marriages follow one of the Christian traditions, although many are atheist or non-religious in general. There are many women, religious or not, who find this sort of relationship to be ideal, and are the ones to bring it up in the first place.

There is an emphasis on sexually monogamous relationships, including the condemnation of pornography. Marriage, or at least long-term, committed relationships, are also important to the Taken in Hand philosophy.

Terms associated with Taken in Hand

- Husband - the person who has the authority in the relationship (specific only to Taken in Hand relationships)
- Wife - the person who cedes authority in a Taken in Hand relationship (specific only to this style of relationship).

Female Led Relationships

Female Led Relationships, (FLR), are relationships where the woman is in charge or has the authority in a consensual power exchange. FLR refers to a specific philosophy, not just any relationship where the woman leads. This is a style of relationship between a dominant woman and a submissive man, adhering to a set of rules and levels.

These relationships also include many BDSM activities, including chastity and cuckolding. FLRs are often referred to as “role reversals”, buying into the patriarchal, male-led relationship idea that can be pervasive in society.

Much of the kink seems to be male-centred and male-driven (rather than mutually enjoyed activities that are seen in most F/m relationships). A lot of the writing that can be found on FLRs online include ways to convince your wife to take control or how to encourage a woman into this sort of relationship. Consent is stressed, as is open communication between partners. These things are formalized in a contract for many adherents to FLRs.

Terms associated with FLRs;

- Level 1, Low Key FLR - where the woman is assuming a small amount of control, mostly to please her man and not because she actually wants to.
- Level 2, Moderate FLR - where the woman is willing to take some control but is uninterested in kink or punishment.
- Level 3, Formal FLR - the woman takes control of the “5 food groups” and is willing to participate in kink and punishment. She often takes a more motherly role towards the man.
- Level 4, Extreme FLR - this seems to be the only level where the woman actually enjoys BDSM activities. She sees the ‘benefits’ of a power exchange relationship and it is what she wants.

- 5 Food Groups - the idea that people can negotiate control over 5 key areas of life; free time, finances, household chores, life direction, and sex.

Kink Specific Roles

These roles are specific to certain kinks and may not be as commonly recognized within the greater BDSM community.

Age Play

Age play is where participants take on the behaviours of an earlier age, usually from infancy to young teens. Touted by many as a form of escapism or a way to forget the cares of the real world, some see it as an identity all on its own.

Elements of age play are also used in some relationships, such as Daddy Dom & little girl, which are very popular as of late. The themes of direct age play may not always be obvious, but the parental, nurturing aspect is an important focus of these relationships.

Some people feel that age play should not be sexual in any manner. These are often people who regress or feel that their little side is an innate part of their identity (although some do engage in sexual play during regression). Others enjoy the taboo nature of age role play and sexual activity together.

It should also be noted that while many littles are submissive, it is not something inherent to the role. There are dominant littles and submissive caregivers. Some people enjoy age play without any power exchange at all.

Roles associated with age play include;

- Little - a person who role plays or regresses to a younger age, usually anywhere from an infant to early teens. These are adults who enjoy acting and indulging in things from childhood.
- Middle - a person who role plays or regresses to a younger age, but a bit older than is typical with littles. They will take on characteristics of a child from around 8 years old to teenager.
- Big - the adult partner in an age play scenario
- Daddy Dom - a (usually) male Dominant who prefers a nurturing and paternal role. They may or may not be directly involved in age play as DDlg (Daddy Dom/little girl) is currently a popular kink. Also a male caregiver for a little.
- Mommy Domme - a female Dominant who prefers a nurturing and maternal role. The term usually refers to the caregiver partner in an age play relationship or arrangement.
- Caregiver - the person who maintains their adult mindset in age play and looks after a little. May or may not be Dominant. Often called Mommy or Daddy by the little.

- AB/DL (Adult Baby/Diaper Lover) - an umbrella term that covers people who role play or regress to an infant's mindset and/or people who enjoy wearing diapers. A person may regress without wearing diapers (although it's rare for someone to be specifically into adult baby play without also being into diapers). Alternately, a person may get a sexual thrill from wearing diapers without any form of age regression.
- Baby Girl - a (usually) female submissive who prefers a nurturing and parental Dominant. They may or may not be involved in age play or age regression.
- Baby Boy - a male submissive who prefers a nurturing and parental Dominant.

Primals

Primals are people who connect to the more primitive and animalistic aspects of humanity during sexual play (or occasionally non-sexual play). Many primals say this is not a role play but an identity. Often referred to as "the beast", or similar by those involved. Identification with wolves (and the debunked hierarchy of wolf families) is common, as is a connection with other powerful animals. It is not animal role play, but taking on real or perceived aspects of those animals.

Primals often describe this state of being as instinctual. Some become non-verbal, or communicate by grunts, growls, or single, snarled words. Some describe acting on instinct, without having to think an action through.

While there is generally a power exchange element to primal play, it is more of a fight or struggle for dominance (even if everyone knows who is supposed to win). Some primals do play without a power exchange element as well.

Some roles associated with primals are;

- Primal Predator - a person who enjoys consensually hunting, taking down, and physically overpowering their partner.
- Primal Prey - a person who wants to be consensually hunted, taken down, and physically overpowered. Will often fight back hard against this happening, similar to resistance play.

Sexual Play

This section covers a wide variety of sexual practices, from multiple partners to chastity. Specific kinks are also loosely defined here, more detail will be given in the Exploring Sexual Taboo chapter.

Cuckolding/cuckqueaning usually involves one partner sleeping with someone outside the relationship and using this to humiliate or degrade their partner. All aspects are consensual, and the person being cuckolded is often the initiator of the scenario. The outside sexual partner will often participate in the humiliation as well.

Cuckolding/cuckqueaning can also involve race play and fetishism, an aspect that some are uncomfortable with. The stereotype that black men are better endowed and have more raw sexual power comes into play often in these scenarios. It can be difficult terrain to navigate without crossing the line into benevolent (or not) racism.

Hotwifing involves a man sharing his wife with others consensually and without humiliation. Her sexual prowess may be a point of pride for him or he may be demonstrating his dominance by ordering her to sleep with his friends. There may or may not be an aspect of power exchange in a hotwife scenario.

Both cuckolding/cuckqueaning and hotwifing can involve the partner being witness to the outside sexual activity, or they may be told about it before or after the fact, usually in detail.

Chastity play involves the denial of sex and masturbation, sometimes with the use of chastity devices. This is a kink that plays out well when partners have to be in different locations, as a way of eroticising that distance and inability to have physical sex.

Swinging is where couples swap partners for sex. It is not kink activity, but some swingers also explore kink, while some kinksters explore swinging. Traditionally the two communities do not get along, due to differences in cultural norms and accepted behaviour. There is some cross-over since many swing clubs host kink or fetish nights.

Roles associated sexual kinks include;

- Cuckold - the male partner of a “cheating” woman, who enjoys being humiliated while his wife/female partner has sex with other men. He may be witness or participate in the play by acting as a “fluffer” for either/both partners. Some wish to perform oral sex on their female partner after she has sex with the bull.
- Bull - the man who is having sex with the female partner of a cuckold. He may also contribute to the humiliation of the cuckold or may not wish to be involved in that aspect.
- Cucktress - the woman having sex with the bull.
- Cuckquean - a woman whose male partner has sex with other women to humiliate her. The female version of a cuckold.
- Hotwife - the female partner in a hetero relationship who has sex with other men for her own sexual enjoyment and because it turns her partner on. There is no aspect of humiliation involved.
- Keyholder - the person who is holding the key to a chastity device, and controlling access to the genitals of the person wearing it. Usually the dominant partner, who decides how long the chastity will last.

- Sensual Dominant - a dominant (or often a top) who engages in mostly or entirely sensual and sensation based play, with very little, if any, pain play.
- Slut - a person of any gender who enjoys sexual play. May or may not have multiple partners.
- Swinger - a person involved in swinging. Someone who swaps partners with another couple for sexual play.

Animal & Pet Play

This type of play involves a person who takes on the characteristics and mannerisms of an animal. They will role play as that animal for the duration of the scene. Many people feel an intense connection with the animal they choose. It is often used as a way to escape stressful human existence, where one can become an animal and not have to worry about the things that people have to deal with, at least for a short time.

Animal & pet play may or may not involve sexual activity. Some people are completely turned off by the idea and others enjoy the taboo aspect.

Many participants enjoy elaborate costumes and gear, to help them get into the animal mindset.

Animal and pet play can involve elements of power exchange or it may be done without any form of power exchange. People often engage in this sort of play alone, without a partner.

Roles associated with animal & pet play include;

- Furry - a person who dresses up and takes on the mannerisms of an animal. Often wears a full fursuit, which can resemble a plushie or stuffed toy. Distinct from pet play.
- Pony - a person who acts like a horse or pony and wears items like reins, bits, blinders, shoes with hooves, and tails to look more like a horse or pony.
- Trainer - a person who trains a human animal in various activities
- Handler - a person who is in charge of a human animal, offering training, affection, and other things the human animal may need.
- Pet - a human animal that is generally pampered by their owner
- Owner - a person who owns a human pet. Usually dominant.
- Pup/Puppy - a person who takes on the mannerisms of a dog or puppy. Often associated with gear such as puppy masks, tails, paws and collars.
- Kitten - a person who takes on the mannerisms of a cat or kitten. Less emphasis on the gear, but ears and a tail are common.

Other Roles

These are the roles that didn't fit into any of the above categories.

- Brat - a person who enjoys pushing the buttons of their partner, to elicit play or harsher play. Many have a bad reputation for engaging in this sort of boundary-pushing behaviour with people who have not consented to it. A somewhat controversial role in BDSM communities
- Pixie - a person who enjoys playful teasing of their partner or banter while playing. Usually done to get a laugh or to encourage funishment.
- Cross-dresser - a person who wears clothing traditionally associated with the opposite gender for sexual or other gratification. The person does not identify as that gender (although they may take on a name appropriate for that gender while they are dressed). It is a role play, not to be confused with people who are transgender, which is an identity.
- Deviant - a person who does not conform to society's expectations of them, either through appearance, life choices, attitude, or in any other way.
- Disciplinarian - a person, usually dominant, who doles out discipline, often in the form of corporal punishment.
- Doll - a person who transforms their outward appearance to look more doll-like. Also, a person who enjoys being treated as a doll, including objectification.
- Exhibitionist - a person who enjoys performing sexual acts where others will see, to elicit a reaction.
- Financial Dominant - a person whose kinks involve money and the power aspects of giving, taking, or controlling money.
- Fin Domme - a woman who engages in kinks surrounding money as the dominant partner, often as a means of income.
- Looner - a balloon fetishist
- Newbie - a person who is new to BDSM
- Pay Pig - a person who submits to a financial dominant
- Pig - a person who is really into a certain type of play, ie pain pig. Also, someone who indulges in dirty play that may involve mud, dirt, oil, sweat, or things that most people would consider 'nasty'.
- Voyeur - a person who gets sexual pleasure from watching others engage in sex or kink.

Remember, there are many, many roles available to you, this has just been a sampling. Most people will start with the basics - play and power exchange roles - before exploring others. Do what feels right for you and use whichever roles work for you.

6 EXPLORING BDSM:

WARM-UPS IN BDSM PLAY

A theme that you will see repeated through this book (and many others which concern BDSM play) is the idea of a warm up. While there are a few people who prefer not to play with a warm-up, it is generally considered part of good play.

Think about it. When you're having sex, do you jump right from fully clothed to penetrative sex? Sometimes, yeah, you might. Most of the time, however, it's much nicer to take your time, engage in kissing, caressing, and slowly work your way to the main event (if penetrative sex is the main event for you). Even those times when you skip all that stuff, it's usually because you've been teasing each other in different ways - the foreplay has been verbal, for example.

BDSM is no different in this respect. The play is a lot more fun if you start slow or light and work your way up in intensity.

This can be done in a number of ways. If we are talking about impact play, you would start with lighter strokes and toys that are less intense. As you go on, the intensity gets greater. Hits are stronger. The really evil toys come out.

If we are talking about sensation play, it starts out more gentle. Often the goal of sensation play is things which feel good in a sensual or sexual manner, so starting with kissing or caressing may be a good start. Light tickles along the arms, legs or back may be a good way to start a tickle scene, progressing to the belly or feet (or wherever the person is most ticklish).

Wax play may start with very low temp candles held high to lessen the heat, over the back. It could progress to candles being held closer to the skin, slightly higher temp candles or wax being dripped in more intimate places - or all of those!

Even a humiliation scene can follow this progression. It may start with some slight verbal teasing or mild humiliation, progressing through some embarrassing situations and culminating with serious degradation and/or humiliating scenarios.

Bondage often has the warm-up built in, since it takes time to bind someone thoroughly. Likewise, role play often has a warm-up built in as the participants find their character and become more comfortable with them (and lose that "silly" feeling!).

Warm Up & Bottom/Top Space

Bottom space, commonly referred to as subspace, can be a goal for some people during play. If it is, a proper warm-up goes a long way to helping a person achieve this headspace. Similarly, it can also set the rhythms needed to achieve top space.

For those unfamiliar with these concepts, they are a well known but poorly understood phenomenon within BDSM. Without getting into the more controversial ideas about top and bottom space, there has been some limited scientific research done on the subject.

These headspaces are thought to be what's known as a "flow state". Flow state happens in many different disciplines, from sports to the arts. It is when the body and brain become so singularly involved in an activity that a feeling of oneness or peace can be felt. This can be an intense, energetic feeling, as one gets in sports when instinct takes over and the body performs in perfect synchronization with the mind. People often refer to it as "the zone". In art and the various forms of artistic expression, it can be an utter calm full of creativity. Time often seems to melt away and all that matters is what's in front of you.

While I don't purport to describe anyone's feelings of bottom or top space, it can often be a similar feeling in BDSM. The idea that one becomes so immersed in the scene that the outside world melts away. That everything flows perfectly from one moment to the next. For many people, it can be an almost spiritual experience.

There is also the aspect that endorphins play in BDSM, especially for bottoms. Many people will argue that the endorphin high is separate from bottom space, while others say it is an important aspect of it. Some bottoms achieve bottom space during activities which would not involve any endorphins at all.

The words subspace, bottom space, dom space and top space describe a general concept. The experience of that concept is going to be different for each person who, and likely a bit different each time. It's one of those "you'll know it when you feel it" sort of things.

Not everyone who is engaged in BDSM play wants to enter this headspace. Some find they feel less in control and dislike the feeling. Others find they fall too deeply into the role and become too compliant - to the point that they are unable to enforce boundaries or appropriately look after themselves. They may want to experience this feeling with a deeply trusted partner but not during casual play. Others simply don't like the feeling.

The Point of Warm-Ups

Warm-ups are still important if you are uninterested in bottom or top space. They provide a way for the body and mind to acclimatize to the feelings of play. Many of the things we do in BDSM can be jarring to both the body and mind if we just dive right into the deep end. Warm-ups help our bodies and minds get used to what is going to happen.

If you've ever had a spanking where the top just hauls off and hits hard on the first swat, to the point that it hurts and not in the "sexy" way, you know how important warm-ups are. That same swat later on in play, once you're both warmed up and excited might feel perfect - or not hard enough!

By starting with light swats, the body can relax. Warm up play is usually done in a predictable rhythm, so you know when to anticipate the next swat. The rhythm can be slow, fast, or anything in between as long as it's predictable. This helps the bottom relax and not tense up waiting for a blow that may or may not land (don't worry, if you like playing like that, it's fine to do later on!).

Warm-ups aren't just for bottoms, tops benefit from them too. Has your hand ever gotten sore not even halfway through a planned spanking, causing you to stop or reach for a paddle you didn't intend to use? Warm-ups will help prevent this. It's literally the same, in this case, as the bottom's bottom. You warm up the skin, getting it used to the impact. I've done bare handed spankings without a break for an hour or more, all because I did a proper warm up.

Warm-ups also provide a time for connective touch. By rubbing, caressing, and generally incorporating some gentle contact, it can make the scene feel more intimate while providing important information to the top.

A top will want to pay attention to things like skin temperature. This light play will literally warm up the skin as blood rushes to the surface because of the stimulation. In lighter skinned bottoms, you will be able to see this as well, as the skin becomes a lovely shade of pink. You may have to look a little more closely to see this in darker skinned bottoms, especially in the dim lighting that is popular in many dungeons. By feeling the warmth of the skin, you get the same feedback without the need for visual confirmation (and it can be handy for tops who are visually impaired or just not wearing their glasses).

Touching the bottom's skin will also allow you to check them over for any bruises or other, minor injuries that could interfere with your play. Are there some bruises left over from the last scene you did together? Playing in the same area isn't a big deal but it will be more prone to bruising this time around, so it's important to be aware.

Connective touch and light swats can also help the bottom become accustomed to your touch. It doesn't matter if you've just met or been married for 50 years, allowing another person to touch us can be an intimate experience. Hopefully, it will be exciting, maybe sensual, maybe sexually arousing. Warm-ups can give you both (all) a chance to get into the mood, especially if you haven't engaged in any pre-play rituals.

When we are talking about play that involves humiliation or other forms of emotional sadism/masochism, starting out slow and doing a warm up - even if there is no physical contact - will give you a chance to get into the right headspace. So for a top, it allows them to access that part of themselves that can be cruel when needed and turn off the filters required for most social situations. For bottoms, it can help them get into a place where they can take the shame and humiliation that is about to happen and process it as a positive experience.

A lesser-known reason to engage in a warm-up is that it can minimize marking. Now, there is a point where skin will bruise no matter how much warming up you've done. So if you're a fan of marks, don't worry! As a professional Dominatrix, I played with a lot of people who could not have marks left from play, for a variety of reasons. I learned quickly that a proper warm-up would allow me to play more intensely with a bottom for whom marks were an issue.

Pre-Scene Rituals

We will discuss protocol as a form of play and ways to reinforce your dynamic later on in Exploring Protocols & Power Exchange. For now, I do want to touch on opening rituals because they can be a part of your warm up.

An opening ritual is designed to help you get into the right headspace. It, like other protocols in BDSM, will help establish a power dynamic. It can be used to indicate the beginning and end of a scene.

This is especially helpful if your relationship is bedroom only and otherwise egalitarian. Placing boundaries around the scene by using a ritual makes it clear when the power exchange starts and stops. Even if you have a full time power exchange dynamic, having a clear beginning and end to your play can be helpful.

Rituals are personal and should be adjusted to fit your dynamic. However, there are some simple things which can work for many different people and dynamics. Feel free to add, take away or scrap the whole thing altogether. Find what works for you if this doesn't feel right.

Of course, like most elements of BDSM, opening rituals are entirely optional, so if this idea doesn't speak to you, don't use it.

My Opening Ritual for Play

I will start with having the bottom kneel in the centre of the play space where I can walk around them if I choose to. If they can't kneel, I will have them seated on a stool. Pretty much anything that brings their head lower than mine and where I can have them exposed and feeling vulnerable.

I may have them naked or mostly undressed at this point, or I may allow them clothing, if I have plans for that later (or if the scene demands, or if it's one where the clothes stay on, etc.). If they are naked, I expect that clothing will be folded neatly and placed in a corner or under the cross, somewhere out of the way. I always check on the folded neatly part. You would be amazed at how many people ignore that part of my orders or just don't know how to fold clothing. If you need/want an excuse for funishment, this is a good one!

I won't say anything other than giving orders or corrections. If this is someone I've been playing for a while, I expect them to know what to do. If they're new to me, I will give detailed instructions, but only for so long, I expect them to learn after a few repetitions/scenes. Correcting them on any part of this ritual/protocol can also serve as a good reason for funishment, especially for those who find training and ritualized BDSM to be a turn on.

My silence or relative silence during this time can be unnerving to the bottom. I want it to be this way. While they're feeling self-conscious or fumbling due to nervousness, I like to casually sit, legs crossed and watch them like a hawk. I want them to see me watching them. I want them to feel my eyes on them the whole time. I also want them to see how relaxed I am compared to how tense they are. I want them to know that I am in charge, without having to say a thing.

I may grab a toy like a crop to use for corrections and to direct them. It's that classic Dominatrix look but it works for people of any gender. It's handy to have something that I can use to give a swat without having to get up. Something I can use to get their attention by placing it under their chin. Something that makes a good noise if I'm especially displeased and feel the need to abruptly get their attention.

Once they are undressed (if applicable) and kneeling (or in the correct position), I want to make them feel even more unbalanced mentally and vulnerable. I will have them kneel upright (not resting their buttocks on their heels), with arms behind their head like prisoner or behind their back, out of the way. It means that they can't use their hands to cover nakedness or to balance. Both are positions associated with being a captive of some sort.

Don't be afraid to use silence and inaction during this time to build tension. They don't know what's going to happen next. Or they might, if you've done this ritual with them before, but either way drawing it out can help reinforce that you're in charge and they aren't.

Next, I like to do an inspection of my property. This is exactly what it sounds like. I will walk around the bottom, inspecting every inch of their body. Now, I've played with a huge variety of people, from those who were not very confident in their bodies to those who loved their bodies. I learned, very quickly, that we all have hangups about our bodies. Even the people who look like Greek gods and goddesses.

As long as this isn't a sore spot for your bottom (and let's face it, many people have body issues that we don't want to make worse), go over every inch. Don't say anything (unless you're both into that type of humiliation - I'm not). Just looking with a neutral expression is enough to get most people feeling pretty uncomfortable. Only touch for corrections in posture or pose and use the crop to do it, not your hand. I like to go for "cold and aloof" during this part.

For extra oomph, you may want to have the bottom switch positions to all fours or another, very exposed position. Have them spread their legs or ass cheeks so you can get a better look at their genitals or asshole. If they weren't feeling like an object owned by you by this point, this should do the trick.

At this point, I will place their play collar around their neck and fasten or lock it. Even within my long-term relationships, I will have a play collar for my partner, even though they are always my submissive. Play collars are usually the spiked, leather dog collars that are often associated with BDSM play. They generally aren't acceptable to wear day to day, even for us "alternative" folks. For casual play, I have a few play collars that I can choose from, not nearly as nice as the ones I've bought for serious partners.

Once the collar is in place, I like to have them show a little appreciation. For a regular partner, I may want a kiss. For a casual partner, kissing my shoes may be more appropriate. Of course, if your partner is into feet/shoes, it may be a nice reward for passing inspection.

Things to Think About

Go over the elements of this ritual in your mind. Picture it playing out the way I've written it. Now, ask yourself a few questions;

- What sort of mood or tone does this ritual set?
- How can I change that mood, while keeping with the spirit of what's written?
- What is the significance of each part? Why would I do these things, in this order?
- Which parts do you find to be the most important?

Let's take a look at answering a few of these.

Obviously, the mood or tone set is a more serious one. It plays into the stereotype of the cold, strict dominant. It reinforces the idea that my partner is simply an object, one that may please me, but one that will have to work to earn my praise. It shows that I am in charge, that I will correct any behaviour I don't like, that bad behaviour will be punished and good will be rewarded.

That tone is fine for some play scenes, but what if you want something more light-hearted and loving? Ice Queen (or King) isn't your thing, you prefer Love Goddess/God.

That's okay, we will need to skip to the last question first, though. What parts are the most important? The collar is the big one. When it goes on, playtime starts. When it comes off, play time is over. It gives us a definitive start and finish point for the dynamic, as well as a constant reminder during the scene. The concept of one person being in power while another serves is also important to this ritual.

So let's turn the Ice Queen into a more benevolent ruler. Rather than being silent, give gentle direction and praise when the bottom is obedient. Forget the crop, use your hands. If you like the idea of a prop, choose something more sensual that will feel nice against the skin. Touch your partner, caress their skin.

When you do the inspection, tell them how appealing they look to you. You may choose to tease them with ideas of what's to come in the scene, or just leave it open-ended. "Oh, what I will do to you..." can say a lot without really saying anything. Show delight in their body and their reactions when you touch them. Comment positively on any outward signs of arousal.

When you place the collar around their neck, maybe choose one that feels nicer. Leather and steel spikes are awesome, but in this case, maybe fur lined or silky is better. Rather than locking it in place as a sign of them being owned property, lovingly placing it around their neck as if it's a prize can drastically change the mood.

Finish up with a long, slow, deep kiss or other show of loving affection. If they do enjoy body worship, indulge them in a gentle way.

You can see how these changes can completely change the tone and expectations for the scene to come. It still follows the same basic script, has similar actions, but the intentions are different. Things that were used to unnerve can easily be turned into things to show appreciation.

Before we move on to our checklists and scenes, think about a few things. You can write them down here, or make a copy of this page and keep track there.

What elements do you think are important to have in an opening ritual?

What mood do you like to set before a play scene? Which moods are most common for your play style? If you're totally new, what mood do you fantasize about the most?

How many different moods can you set by changing small elements of this ritual?

What can you do to evoke those moods in an opening ritual, either by altering mine here or creating your own?

7 EXPLORING BDSM:

AFTERCARE

Aftercare in BDSM is the time spent after your play scene, usually cuddling, talking or even eating. It's a chance for people to have some intimate downtime together, enjoying the feelings that play has brought them and is a valuable bonding time for the couple.

Aftercare also provides a more practical purpose. It is widely believed that aftercare can lessen or even totally negate drop after a scene. It allows participants to return to their regular state of mind and deal with any emotional issues that the scene may have brought up.

This is especially important to those just starting out or people doing more intense scenes. Often when we play we are taking on a persona that is slightly or drastically different than who we are. Even if we remain ourselves for the duration of the scene, we access a part of ourselves that we don't usually allow to come out. This can leave us feeling very vulnerable. For some tops, it can leave them feeling like a monster.

Drop

A lot has been written and talked about when it comes to sub-drop or bottom drop. Less talked about dom or top drop. Both of these can cause distress if not dealt with in a proper and timely manner. The problem is knowing what causes it and what will help it in your specific case.

It is thought that drop is caused by the sudden drop in endorphins or other hormones that are released during a play scene. Drop can feel like a deep sense of exhaustion, disorientation, or sadness. You may feel cold and have a hard time getting warm again. People will sometimes report feeling not quite themselves, without being able to pinpoint what exactly is wrong. Some people will feel ravenously hungry. Others may cry at the drop of a hat, or for no reason at all.

Drop isn't always the result of play. People who attend conventions for leisure activities are familiar with con-drop, the feeling of sadness that often happens when you leave and go back to the real world. You've spent a few days in a space that is full of other people who are into the same thing as you, made new friends, had a blast and now there is nothing but the mundane day to day. This happens with BDSM conventions and can even happen after smaller kink events.

Of course, not everyone experiences drop or drops with every scene. It is one of those things that you won't know affects you until it does. You could play 100 times and be fine, but on the 101st time, drop hits you. You may experience it the first time you play and never again. No one knows how they will react to something new, so it's best to be prepared. If you know enough to look out for the signs of drop, then you can have strategies in place to help fix it.

Most of the time, drop will resolve within a few hours of play. You tend to the needs that you and your partner(s) have, and start to feel better. For some people, no special aftercare is needed. For others, they have elaborate rituals that they perform after play, to ward off drop and to help ease them back into the real world after living a fantasy for a short time.

The most important thing to remember when dealing with drop is to communicate to your partner(s) when you aren't feeling 100% after a scene. If you're feeling out of sorts, it's best to alert your partner so that they can look for signs you may be experiencing drop and do what they can to prevent it from getting worse. Even the act of talking about it can ease some types of drop. For instance, if you're feeling down after a scene, talking to your partner about it can go a long way to making you feel better.

Finally, it is important to know that drop doesn't always happen right after the scene. It can happen a few hours or even a few days after your scene. If you wake up a day or two later feeling a bit down, it could be drop. Many tops like to check on their partner a few days after the scene (if they aren't already in regular communication) for this very reason.

Types of Aftercare

Aftercare can be broadly placed into two categories; physical and emotional. Each one provides for different needs a person may have after a scene. While these lists are far from exhaustive, they may serve to give you ideas for what you may need after you're done exploring. If you need something that isn't on the list, ask for it.

I should point out that while some people see removing ropes/restraints and cleaning up the play space as aftercare, I simply see them as part of the regular practice of play. As a top and a dominant, I do find that cleaning the toys at the end of a scene is a bit of time to collect myself, a small ritual where I can simply focus on such a simple task.

Physical Aftercare

Taking care of any first aid which needs to be done. While this should be done over the course of the scene, sometimes dressing wounds from play piercings, for instance, could be part of aftercare.

- Sharing some food or drink. Have a glass of water, a cup of tea, a few cookies or some fruit. I love to get a good meal after playing, it's hard work that takes a lot of energy!
- Snuggling up in a warm blanket or wrapping your partner in a warm blanket.
- Cuddling in a quiet place.
- Take a short nap.
- Talk about the scene, the weather, pretty much anything!
- Kissing, caressing, even sexual activity is a favourite of many people.
- Massage or other relaxing activities.
- Have a shower, together or separate.
- Watch television or a movie together.
- Pretty much anything else you can think of!

Emotional Aftercare

- Talk about the scene. This won't be an in-depth debrief, but more like a casual conversation about how much fun it was.
- Reassure your partner. If humiliation was a part of the scene, you may need to reassure your partner that those things you said weren't true. Likewise, if a scene involved heavy sadism, you may need to reassure your partner that they aren't a monster!
- Hold your partner while they cry. Some scenes are meant to elicit strong emotions. Some are meant to bring about catharsis. If either of these things happens (and even if they don't) your partner may be overwhelmed by emotion. In this case, it's best to let it out and just hold them, offering reassurance as needed.
- Any other form of emotional support you can offer your partner.

Any of these types of aftercare are totally acceptable, as are things which are not on the list. If you know you need or prefer aftercare, that is something that should be talked about during negotiations. If you are unsure if aftercare is something you might need, you should express that during your scene negotiation. It's okay to be new and unsure if you will need something or not. A good partner will accept this and make arrangements to either provide aftercare if you think you may need it or to have someone available that you can turn to if you need.

No Aftercare

Some people don't like aftercare. This doesn't make them bad or wrong, it just means that they're not into it. People are individuals and not everyone will like the same things.

I find that aftercare is often too intimate for me when it comes to casual play. I also avoid cuddling with anyone other than intimate partners, because I have chronic pain and any touch can feel like knives stabbing into my body. My partners know where and how to touch me to lessen that pain, a more casual partner may not.

Some bottoms do not like aftercare. They just want to enjoy the 'glow' of the pain alone. They may prefer to process things on their own. They may just not want to be touched. There is any number of reasons that a person may not want to be involved with aftercare. This is okay, but it should be talked about during negotiations.

Of course, when I say people who don't do aftercare, I mean those who aren't into the general style of cuddles, blankets, and sweet words. A responsible player will tend to any first aid needs, get their partner a glass of water if they need it, and have a bit of a chat after play. They aren't going to just pack up toys or put on clothing and walk away without saying a word. A good kinkster will ensure that their partner is okay before wandering off to rejoin the party or do something else.

If you are planning on playing with someone who doesn't do aftercare, but you need it, there are options. You can have a surrogate for aftercare. A friend who is happy to provide any emotional or physical aftercare that you may need after a scene, from cuddling to crying.

Self Care

You can also practice self-care or self-administered aftercare.

The world of kink can be funny sometimes. Tops and dominants have been practising self-care after scenes for as long as anyone can remember. We are just expected to bounce back and not have negative emotions or reactions to scenes. Obviously, this isn't true for all people all of the time, so tops and dominants learned the art of self-care.

More recently, this idea of self-care for bottoms and submissives started getting talked about. Some were like "we've been doing that since forever!" and others found it to be an almost revolutionary thing.

Either way, self-care after a scene can help prevent drop and help to maintain a happy and healthy approach to BDSM. It is an important skill to learn if you are interested in pick up or casual play at parties since many people are more reluctant to share an intimate moment after play with someone they don't know that well. Think of it like sex; when having sex with a long-term partner, you cuddle after or talk with each other. During a one night stand or casual partner situation, the cuddling may be kept to a minimum.

Some things that you may want to do as a form of self-care after a scene

- Have a warm blanket to cuddle up in.
- Have a first aid kit and manual available, in case something comes up after the fact.
- Have a bubble bath or enjoy a bath with scented oils or a bath bomb.
- Relax with a scented candle or incense.
- Read your favourite book, watch your favourite movie or TV show.
- Have some hard candy or chocolate.
- Have a light or hearty meal - comfort food is optional!
- Enjoy a hot cup of tea or a glass of wine (or any other beverage that you like).
- Write in a private journal. (Note: it is best not to write publicly, like a blog, right after play. Your emotions may be off kilter and you don't want to post something you will regret later. If you must, write but wait a day or two to publish).
- Cuddle with your favourite stuffed animal.
- Write a letter to your partner, or have them write one for you that you can read if you drop at a time when they can't be reached.
- If you also identify as a little, get out the crayons and colouring books.

Don't forget that both or all partners can be in an altered state of mind after playing. It is best to allow enough time to come down before engaging in activities that require a lot of focus, like driving. A person after play can be just as impaired as a person who has had a few drinks. Make sure you are in the right frame of mind before you get behind the wheel or do anything else. This includes making public posts on social media or texting your ex!

8 EXPLORING BDSM:

PUNISHMENT VS FUNISHMENT

In the chapter on common mistakes, we will speak about the definitions of words and how they can be different to different people. Within the world of BDSM, there seems to be a huge misuse of the word punishment.

Punishments are a penalty that is imposed on a person who disobeys. The person may disobey the law and go to jail as punishment. They may disobey an order in the military and be court-martialed. They could disobey the unspoken rules of society and be ostracized as punishment. Within a power exchange relationship, they could disobey the rules they agreed to follow and be made to write lines, endure an activity they hate, or any number of other punishments.

Funishments, on the other hand, are those things we find enjoyable. Many people find the idea of punishment erotic, they want to be punished because they enjoy it. Maybe they enjoy the idea that something they do is so scandalous, they would be punished for it, all the while loving the humiliation that goes along with the scenario. There are as many ways to enjoy or erotocise punishment as there are people who love it.

The big difference is that funishments are for fun, not for an actual breaking of the rules. Punishments are reserved for those times when everyone involved agrees it's time.

If you choose to have rules in your relationship (see Exploring Protocol & Power Exchange, you will make rules that have meaning to you and your partner(s). Most people feel that it's painful to know your partner knowingly broke one of your agreements. This may be a time when punishments are appropriate. We separate out funishments because we wouldn't want our partners to cause this sort of hurt to indicate they want to play.

While you don't need an excuse to engage in funishment, some people enjoy the dynamic of brats. A brat may push the dominant/top's buttons, doing things which are playful rather than hurtful to garner a funishment. Gentle teasing is a great example. It can be fun to banter back and forth with your partner, then take them over your knee when the time seems right.

Contrast that scenario with a partner who agreed to a "no talking back" rule but constantly breaks it in hope that you will punish them. In this case, not giving play would be the most cruel punishment. Furthermore, in this scenario, if you were to punish said partner, you would only be rewarding the behaviour you want to eliminate.

For this reason, nearly every person who engages in a punishment dynamic will say that you should never use play activities as punishments. So if you and your partner enjoy spanking for fun it should *never* be used as a punishment. It sends the wrong message and is simply too confusing to maintain.

If you are interested in using punishments in your dynamic, make sure that they are unpleasant things. Obviously, they need to be consensual, but they shouldn't be enjoyable. Just like when we were young, you can use many of the same punishments now. Loss of privileges can really hurt. Imagine not being allowed to log into your social media accounts for a week? Or not being able to indulge in your favourite hobby as punishment.

A popular - and more constructive - punishment that is fairly common within punishment dynamics is to have the person being punished write an essay. They would need to write about what rule they broke, the purpose of the rule, and details on how they will work to correct their behaviour. The idea here is that introspection is needed to correct unwanted behaviour.

Whatever you decide to use as punishments, the rules and expectations should be laid out clearly in the beginning. There should be a grace period for learning the rules or slowly introducing the rules, allowing time for them to sink in. We will look more closely at creating rules in the Exploring Protocol and Power Exchange chapter.

If you prefer funishments and like to have an excuse, making "playtime rules" that can be broken without any genuine disappointment or hurt can be a good strategy. Rules like using an honorific, no talking back, counting cane strokes and thanking the top after each one is a great way for a bottom to rack up more and more funishment.

Either way, it's important to be on the same page. You wouldn't want a partner who acts out in hurtful ways because they think it's how to initiate play. You wouldn't want to have bad behaviour reinforced because it's rewarded with pleasurable activities. Having an honest conversation and making sure you are defining things the same way will help avoid these mishaps.

9 EXPLORING BDSM: TYPICAL FIRST TIME MISTAKES (AND HOW TO AVOID THEM)

When you're brand new to something, you're bound to make mistakes. It's one of those things you should be okay with before you start experimenting. You're going to make mistakes and that's okay! Learn from them, handle them appropriately and grow. That's how we become well-rounded people.

That said, it seems silly for countless people to endlessly repeat the same mistakes, over and over again. One of the great things about humans is that we are capable of learning from other people's mistakes as well as our own. Understanding why and how someone else has stumbled can help you avoid the same pitfalls.

Too Many Things at Once

This is the first of a few similar mistakes that new people often make. In this case, we are talking about trying to fit too many things at once into a play scene. I know, there are all these fun sounding and interesting things that you've been introduced to, you want to do all of them right away!

If you try to jam too many different activities into a single play scene you're going to end up overwhelmed. You will be fumbling, trying to remember all the things you wanted to do and waste valuable time worrying about whether you did them all. This will interrupt the flow of the scene, damage your confidence, and not be much fun for anyone involved.

Avoid this mistake by selecting between 2 and 5 activities that you want to do. 5 is probably too many activities for some scenes, but it really depends on what they are. If you're doing an impact scene, selecting 5 different styles of implement seems reasonable. On the other hand, if you decide you want to do electrical play, sounding, an elaborate shibari tie, forced orgasms, and fire cupping...well, you will quickly find yourself in trouble.

The problem with the above scenario is that each of those activities takes a while. There is a lot of set up for an activity like sounding, for instance. Elaborate shibari ties can take half an hour or more to complete. The set up that you need to safely do fire cupping is different than the set up to do the bondage or sounding. You can see how you would end up with a scene that lasts hours but is mostly spent setting up for the next activity.

The other problem is that the scene can become disjointed. Ideally, you want to have activities that work together or flow from one to the next. Shibari and wax play are a traditional combination. Bondage with cuffs, rope, or leather restraints can work with just about any activity or it can be the star of the show. You will learn which activities work best together based on your own personal style (as you develop it) and what you observe others doing.

Frenzy

Frenzy is something that happens to many, if not most, people who are new to BDSM. A whole new world is open to you and you want to experience all of it. Right now. What are we waiting for?

While that's not always a big deal on its own, frenzy becomes dangerous when people start playing above their experience level. If you're brand new, doing edge play without any instruction is dangerous. Tops won't have the skills they need and bottoms may not be ready to cope with the emotions it can bring up or fully understand the risks. Many have been known to intentionally disregard the risks because they are chasing that 'high' that all these new activities can bring. Pair these well-intentioned but inexperienced new people together and it's a disaster waiting to happen.

Avoid this mistake by understanding that frenzy happens and it's totally normal. Ask just about any kinkster you know, it's likely happened to them. By being aware of frenzy and knowing to look for the signs, you can protect yourself and your partner.

You may even want to set some ground rules for yourself about how to pace yourself and what limits you want to stick to. Decide that you aren't going to try anything new until you've had a chance to research it and understand the risks. I always encourage both tops and bottoms to attend workshops on the activities they are looking to try. Sometimes you can try it out at the workshop with the help of the instructor. Even if you don't, you will still learn valuable lessons. You will have a basis to develop that skill and you will be able to better recognize who is a safe player and who isn't.

Overconfidence

Many people walk into the world of BDSM thinking that it all looks easy. I mean, how hard can it be to hit people with a stick or wrap them up in ropes?

The answer is that there's a lot to learn. Yes, some activities are pretty straightforward. Spanking is pretty simple when you think about it, but even then, you would be amazed at how many people mess it up. Warm-ups are important to enjoyable impact play - don't worry, we will talk all about them in the appropriate section - without one, enjoyable pain can turn into annoying pain very quickly.

Avoid this mistake by being humble. Many things aren't as easy as they look. Before you engage in an activity, read up about it. Take a class if you're able to. Kinksters love attending workshops. Even those of us who have been around a long time still attend various workshops. Even if it's an activity that I know a lot about, I still learn new tips and tricks by seeing how others do it.

No Confidence

You're new and nervous. It's not unusual, we were all new once. I don't think anyone is ever totally confident doing something for the first time, but a bit of nervousness is different than not having any confidence.

If you aren't confident in what you're about to do, you will make mistakes. You will be so worried about not being perfect that you will sabotage yourself. You may forget what comes next, you might totally freeze when giving or getting an order.

Avoid this mistake by doing your research. Attend some classes, munches, and play parties. Watch others and see what aspects you like. Learn everything you can about an activity before trying it on a human.

If you're a top, practice. Pillows are fantastic for practising your aim for impact play. Most of us learned how to use a flogger by hitting pillows. Same for canes, crops, and just about anything you can think of.

Bottoms can prepare too. If you know you're going to be doing bondage, you can do things like yoga that will condition your muscles and keep you flexible. This will help your body cope with the stress of bondage.

Having a Script

It's your first play scene and you know exactly how it should go - right down to what each of you should be saying. If you create a rigid script of each and every thing that's going to happen, you will end up frustrated and you won't have any fun. Things rarely work out exactly as we planned them in BDSM. Without room to improvise, you will be in trouble.

Avoid this mistake by having a general game plan but not a timed out or a scripted idea of what should happen. Knowing that I want to include spanking, flogging, paddling, and caning in a scene is good. Saying I will do 5 minutes of spanking followed by 3 minutes of flogging, then 7 minutes of paddling, back to another 3 minutes of flogging... You get the idea. It's going to be miserable, make everyone unhappy and it doesn't leave any room for the unexpected. What if my partner really hates the paddle I have? Do I subject them to another 6 minutes and 50 seconds of paddling because it's in the script?

A general game plan allows you to be prepared for your scene while still having the flexibility to react when things don't go perfectly. Life rarely goes the way we want it to, so learning to react in a positive way can go a long way to having satisfying scenes.

Your game plan doesn't need to be very detailed, it really depends on you. I may go into a scene knowing that I want to do sensation play; I know I want to use a hood on my partner, some bondage and then go from there. All of my toys are in a dedicated dungeon room, so I have everything I need on hand. Alternately, I may want to do an impact scene at a party. Before leaving home, I grab a bunch of impact toys and some leather restraints. When I get to the party, I will use whatever equipment is available, whether it's a cross or a spanking bench. I restrain my partner then dig into the bag of toys - no further planning needed.

I'm able to play this way because I've been doing BDSM for so long. When you're new, you probably want to plan a bit more. Generally, you want to go from the mildest sensation to the most intense, so knowing what toys give what sensation is important. In the beginning, you may need to think about it, with experience, you know automatically (and can tell just by the materials, shape, etc).

Being Unprepared

Some people will go into a scene with no idea of what they want to do, not even a general plan. While having a script is no good, having no plan is not any better!

If you are unprepared for your scene, you may be stuck thinking about what to do next. You may need to spend time getting the implements that you need - you may even find yourself running from room to room trying to gather everything you need. This can be frustrating for both you and your partner.

Avoid this mistake by having a general game plan before you begin. Gather everything you need in the space that you will be playing in. Think through each element of your scene and make sure you have everything you need in one place. You can even have a bit of pre-scene fun by having your partner lay out the various implements for you - they get a sneak peek at what they will be experiencing once the scene begins, which can build excitement.

If you need something like ice, get that right before you begin. Just get a big glass and fill it with more than you will need. If you need warm water, get a mug of just boiled water, so that it will be the right temperature when you need it.

Don't forget the more mundane things either. Have condoms, gloves, dental dams and lube handy if you will be needing any of those items. Have a blanket or whatever aftercare items you will need within reach. Always make sure you have a first aid kit and other emergency supplies somewhere easy to find.

Not Enough Communication

Talking about our kinks can be hard, especially when you're new. As time goes on, it gets easier and easier, so do your best to get through those first awkward conversations. In the beginning, people will often skip over important points of pre-scene communications, either because they are nervous talking about it or they don't realize it should be discussed.

It is bound to happen, you're in the middle of a scene and something comes up that you haven't talked about yet. Sometimes it's okay to just ask mid-scene and other times it can ruin the mood or even cause the end of the scene. Lack of communication is common, so don't feel bad if (when) it happens to you.

Avoid this mistake by having a conversation about your scene a few days ahead of time. This will give you time to think about things and ask any questions that pop into your mind at 3 am. Some people may even find it's best to plan multiple conversations before the scene, adding a bit to the negotiation each time. Don't forget to go over things the day of the scene - I like to have the final check in right before we start - to make sure nothing has changed and you're still both in the mood for what you discussed.

Not Checking In or Communicating in Scene

Some people think that once they've done the pre-scene negotiation, that's all the communication that's needed. They don't check in as the scene progresses to see where their partner is at and how things are feeling. Since the top is the one doing the actions, it generally falls to them to check in.

Likewise, some bottoms forget that they need to give feedback to the top as the scene plays out. Even if it's just communication by means of moans or grunts, that feedback is important.

Avoid this mistake by checking in with your partner during a scene. You can use the traffic light system (which also covers safe words) of green, yellow, and red. Green means everything is fine, yellow means it's too much, ease up or slow down, and red means stop. It's not unusual to hear "what's your colour" during scenes at a dungeon.

Number scales are also popular for many people. It's a way to measure the intensity of the activity, where 1 is barely feeling anything and 10 is way too intense, stop. This can be helpful for getting used to a partner's pain tolerance or other thresholds. We will talk more about the uses of the number scale in Exploring Impact & Pain Play.

Even if you don't want to use either of these methods, be sure to keep the lines of communication open during your scene. Giving and getting feedback allows you to alter the scene if you need to and ensures that you both (all) enjoy yourselves. Remember, just because we are into BDSM doesn't mean we can read our partner's minds! Using your words is important.

Sky High Expectations

If you've been fantasizing about BDSM for as long as you can remember and you finally get the chance to try it out, you may have some unrealistic expectations. If you go into your first scene expecting that everything will be perfect, you're going to be disappointed. If you expect that your partner can read your mind, you're going to be disappointed.

Avoid this mistake by managing your expectations and learning about the reality of BDSM. There are going to be times when things don't go exactly as planned. Your partner will make mistakes. You will make mistakes. Learn to roll with it, have a laugh if warranted, and keep going.

For instance, I don't think I've ever done a pegging scene where things weren't totally awkward at one point or another. Getting toys and bodies aligned properly can be a challenge (especially when you're short and your partner is more than a foot taller!). Finding the right size toy for that day and moment can take some time. Having hands covered in lube will almost always end in clumsiness. You learn to laugh it off and keep going. If you take yourself too seriously, you won't have any fun at all.

Don't let your fantasy of BDSM cloud the reality of it. I really suggest that people get out to the community and watch others doing scenes - that way you can see first hand that even experienced people can have bloopers from time to time.

Kink as a Competition or Race to Extreme Play

Some people view everything as a competition. They think that they need to be bigger and better than other people. The kink world is no different. There are people who need to show that they are more "hard-core" than the next person by engaging in ever more extreme play.

Others feel that you need to get through this novice stuff like spanking in order to unlock the secrets of extreme play. They see the pictures of bloody bottoms and think "how long until I get there?".

Avoid this mistake by understanding that kink is not a competition. It doesn't matter what anyone else is doing, only what you and your partner(s) are doing. Do you enjoy your play? Then it's perfect. There is no prize for being the most hard-core in the dungeon, so do what makes you happy.

I do understand the appeal of the more extreme parts of BDSM play. I enjoy playing in that style sometimes, when I have a partner who is into it. However, most of the time we do the same things any new person is capable of doing. Extreme scenes take a lot of planning, skill, practice, and often healing time, so they aren't practical to do every week.

If the more extreme end of the kink spectrum appeals to you, take some classes and practice your BDSM skills like negotiation. Understand that many people will want to see that you can handle regular scenes properly before they are willing to explore more dangerous types of play with you. Educate yourself and make sure you aren't getting in over your head.

Not Communicating After a Scene

Wow, another lack of communication mistake? Yep, which really should emphasize how important communication is to BDSM.

The talking doesn't end when the scene does. How will you know if your partner has enjoyed themselves? How will you tell them that the new thing they tried just didn't feel right? Remember, our partners aren't mind readers, so if we want to turn good scenes into great scenes, we need to communicate.

Avoid this mistake by having a debrief when your scene is over. When you discuss things will vary, but you should check in after a scene and find out how it went for each other. Some people will like doing this right after, incorporating it into their aftercare, others prefer to wait a day or two.

Ask questions like "what did you enjoy the most?", "was there anything you didn't like?", "Did you find it kinda awkward when we...?". Share your thoughts and feelings too. Together you can figure out what parts you will want to do again, what you want to do differently and what things you may want to leave out of the next scene.

Using Booze or Recreational Drugs to Calm Nerves

You're nervous before your very first play scene, whether it's with a new partner or your long-term spouse. You may think that it's not such a big deal to reach for that bottle of wine or your stash before you start to play. It will help you calm down, right?

I'm not going to get on some puritan rant here, but mixing intoxicants with play is incredibly dangerous. BDSM has the potential to seriously harm the participants (find me an experienced top who hasn't had a first aid incident or even a trip to the ER). A lot of kink is learning how to do dangerous things in the safest way possible. Part of how we mitigate risks is by being sober when we play.

Avoid this mistake by making a commitment, to your partner as well as yourself, that you won't mix play and intoxicants. It's not just tops who need their wits about them, bottoms need to be able to feel what's happening without dulled senses to communicate safety information. Everyone needs to be sober to consent to play.

I do want to point out that prescription medication is different. You will need to assess on a case by case basis. If you're taking something short term and it's leaving you a little "happy" or drowsy, it may be best to wait until your health situation has resolved. If it's medication you take for a chronic condition, you're probably better with your medication on-board (I know I'm no good without my medication, which I've been taking every day for many years). You know yourself best. Just don't allow your ego to trump safety.

Getting over nerves can be difficult. A time-honoured tip among tops is in the use of blindfolds. A blindfolded bottom can't see how nervous you are. They can't see you fumble with that toy. It can also help the bottom if they are feeling nervous. They don't have to look at the top and feel judged for what they are doing (or what's being done to them).

Sometimes, though, you just need to bite the bullet. You are going to be nervous, we all were at some point. If you can work up the courage to get started, you will find that the nervousness will fade quickly once you start having fun. There are times that jumping in with both feet is appropriate, if you've done your research and negotiation, this may just be that time.

Not Understanding What You're Getting Into

The language of BDSM can be confusing. There are so many new words to learn and definitions can sometimes be...fluid. Your understanding of what something means could be drastically different from what your partner means.

Take the words dom and sub, for instance. While most kinksters agree that those words talk about power exchange there are those who consider them synonymous with top and bottom. Ask a kinky person about edging and one may speak about dangerous play (edge play) while another talks about getting to the point of orgasm then stopping (edging).

So you can see that even if you know the right words to use, you may not be getting your point across as well as you think. Labels should be the starting point for a conversation, not the whole conversation.

Avoid this mistake by always being clear in your communication. Explain what you want and mean in 'long form' rather than just relying on words with dubious definitions. Instead of saying "I'm into spanking" specify whether you're into being hit on the bottom with hands only or if your version of spanking includes the use of paddles and other implements.

This is especially true when it comes to the labels which describe people. Even if we can agree that dominant or submissive are roles within a power exchange relationship, the exact details of those roles can be drastically different between you and me.

10 EXPLORING BDSM:

EXPLORING YOUR FANTASIES

USING THIS BOOK

Maybe you're new to BDSM or maybe you're a seasoned veteran of kinky or sexual exploration. I've designed this book so that you can try things in a methodical manner or you can jump in with both feet, whichever works best for you.

We will look at a number of different types of popular activities within the BDSM realm. If one thing doesn't appeal to you, move on to the next. If one section really speaks to you and you want to try more, stick with it for a while.

Each section will follow the same basic structure. You and your partner will each fill out a BDSM checklist containing some activities within that style of kink. Rate each activity according to how much you enjoy that kink. If you've never done that activity before, rate it based on how much you think you might like it or how highly it rates in your fantasies of things you would like to try.

I highly suggest using a pencil to fill out your checklist, that way you can change your answers after you actually try things. Sometimes, you will end up loving something you weren't sure about. Other times, something you've fantasized about for years will leave you wanting. Sadly, some things make better fantasy than reality. Just about everyone who has played around with BDSM has discovered something they thought was really hot, only to find that the reality didn't live up to the hype.

Now, a lot of things in BDSM take skill and training. I didn't want to limit the lists, I wanted them to be a sample of things you can experience within the world of kink. They are rated, with the easier activities having a star beside them, and things that are much more dangerous or require a lot of forethought and negotiation having a flag. Don't worry about that too much though, there are plenty of things that beginners can have fun with! Think of the other activities as things you can try if the first few times go well and you decide to explore further.

You will also need to indicate if you would like to top or bottom for that activity. Many people enjoy switching or being on the other side of the slash sometimes. You may be dominant but have one or two special things that you enjoy having done to you. As a submissive, you might enjoy performing a service for your dominant by topping them. Kink orientations fit together in a million different ways, find what works for you and try not to worry about rigid roles. Experiment and find out what feels good, physically, emotionally and mentally.

Next, you will want to compare lists with your partner. This is where things get tricky.

With any luck, you will have a few activities that you've both rated highly - a four or five on our scale - with one of you wanting to top and the other to bottom. Maybe you're both into trying both sides, which means you just need to sort out who plays which role first.

Once you figure out those matches, you can start to put a scene together. Pick three or four different things that you have both rated highly and that you think will work well together. These will be the foundation of your scene. Specific advice on scene creation will be offered in each section, along with some examples that you can read through or use to inspire your play.

In some of the sections, there will be additional information on negotiation, relationship styles, or other things you should know when exploring that set of kinks. For instance, when we talk about sexuality and sexual taboos, there are tips on how to negotiate having a third person join you for some sexy fun or how to role play the scenario if you want the fantasy but not the reality. When we talk about protocol and power exchange, you will learn about things specific to authority transfer and how to create a dynamic that works long term.

Of course, this is not simply an academic exercise. You're meant to actually do these things. So the next step is to go and have some kinky fun. Put your plans into action and enjoy. Figure out if you need aftercare and what type. Find out what lives up to the fantasy and what should stay locked in the imagination.

Once you've had a chance to try a few things, give it a couple of days and then sit down and talk about it. Have a scene review or debrief, where you talk about what was good, what wasn't, and why. These conversations can be difficult, especially if you're not used to talking about sex, fantasy, and this sort of intimacy. It is important, though, and will help you develop stronger BDSM relationships. Like negotiation, this type of conversation is a skill and it will get easier with time. I promise.

Once you've tried out a few different sections and you're (hopefully) feeling more confident, I will give my best tips on combining the different elements and creating amazing scenes. This is something that I've been doing for over 20 years now, nearly half of that time as a professional with a full dance card. Take advantage of my years of trial and error while also experimenting and finding what works best for you.

Finally, we will cover how you learn those more dangerous skills, the ones marked with a flag. I always encourage people to get out into the community but I know that's not always an option. I will share different resources you can use to explore and learn, both on your own and within a community setting.

So without further ado, let's get to the fun stuff!

11 EXPLORING IMPACT & PAIN PLAY: SAFETY

As you explore the world of BDSM, you will hear various truths repeated over and over again. A controversial one is that you want to avoid striking the lower back of a person, due to the potential for damage to their kidneys. How true is this? Where is it safe to strike a person? How hard? With which implements? In this chapter, we will answer these questions, so that you can feel comfortable and confident in your impact and pain play, as well as in general BDSM play.

We will start by looking at the best places for impact & pain play on the body. Next, we will explore places that are good but need some precautions. Third, we move on to the areas that should be avoided unless you have specific training or skill in the type of play you want to engage in. Finally, we will look at the places that you should avoid at all times. There are just some places you don't want to go.

The Best Parts to Play On

The best parts of the body to engage in impact and pain play are the ones that are heavily muscled and protected. This includes the upper back, the buttocks, as well as the front and back of the thighs. Let's take a look at each area a little more carefully.

Buttocks

The ass is the hands-down favourite place for impact play by just about every kinkster. It's just such a classic - spanking, paddling, caning, and more are all traditional. It's part of the eroticised idea of punishments that many of us have and play out during our scenes. It's also a safe place to play with heavy impact and pain.

Bums come in many different shapes and sizes, and all are loved in the BDSM world. The thick layers of muscle that give booties their shape also mean that we can go a little wild with the paddles.

Overlapping are the gluteus minimus, gluteus medius, and gluteus maximus. They provide the power to move our legs and work with some smaller muscles to provide stability to the hip joint. The three give a nice, big target to aim for.

At the bottom of each butt cheek, where the maximus ends, there is a place known as the sweet spot. When we stand, the skin folds slightly, protecting it. When bent over a spanking horse or the back of a couch, the sweet spot is exposed. Well aimed strikes to that area will elicit the sweetest screams from a bottom - it's very sensitive. Even if the rest of the buttocks are impervious to your best attempts, the sweet spot delivers the ouch!

Of course, there are a few areas that need to be avoided when playing with a bent over bottom. The tailbone is the most obvious. There is no muscle protection over the tailbone and it can be rather delicate. It's also painful in the bad way to be hit on the tailbone. Make sure your aim is good enough with whatever implement you choose to avoid hitting it. A common precaution is to place a flogger, a thick leather belt or even a folded t-shirt over the lower back and tailbone while playing. It offers a bit of protection and you will know right away if you've missed your mark.

Wrapping the tails of a flogger or the tip of a cane around the hips is also a concern, especially if your bottom has narrower hips. Your blows should be landing in the middle of each cheek and should not wrap. If you find you are getting wrap around the hips, you run the risk of damaging some of the nerves that lie close to the surface. It also just hurts in a very unpleasant manner. You can raise welts and generally leave a bottom unhappy if you're wrapping unintentionally. Practice your aim on a pillow before moving on to a person.

Thighs, Front & Back

While you're having fun spanking your bottom, don't forget to spread the love around a bit. The thighs are another easy and safe spot to play. The back of the thighs are exposed when the bottom is on a spanking horse or bench, or standing at a cross (if you're not playing in a dungeon, they may be bent over the bed or standing against the wall).

The hamstrings cover the back of the thighs in a wonderful display of musculature. Be aware that this is one of the places that women (and those with higher levels of estrogen in their bodies) carry and store fat as well. Fatty areas tend to bruise more easily than muscled areas, so it's important to remember.

Much like the buttocks, the back of the thighs can take a beating. They are pretty tough and desensitized from us sitting, at least when compared to the front of the thighs. Obviously, I'm going to warn against wrapping your implements - unless you're doing it on purpose, it's a sign that you need to go back and practice more. If you are doing it on purpose, I would ask why? Wrapping speeds up the ends of the flogger, cane or other implements, meaning it will do more damage on impact. I have seen a few tops over the years who have mastered wrapping and turned it into an art - but if you're one of them, you're probably not reading an introductory book on BDSM. Stop wrapping and practice more!

You also want to avoid hitting the back of the knee. As we will learn in the "never hit there" section, joints are always a no-go area. No matter how good you are, nothing positive will come from striking joints.

The front of the thighs, protected by the rectus femoris, the vastus medialis, the vastus intermedius, and the vastus lateralis (collectively known as the quadriceps) on the top and outside of the leg, are a wonderful, safe, and surprisingly sensitive place to do impact play. If you move towards the inside of the thigh where the muscles are smaller and generally get less use, you will find a very sensitive spot indeed. Make sure to ease up when you get to the inner thigh, most bottoms won't like the same intensity there are they do on other, tougher parts.

Upper Back

The upper back is covered by an impressive array of muscles. At the top is the Trapezius, which runs from the back of your neck to your shoulder and then onwards to your spine. It's often the muscle targeted when you get a shoulder rub. You won't be hitting much of this muscle when you do impact play on the back, but it's important to note because it helps stabilize everything.

Speaking of shoulders, the deltoid caps the shoulder, meeting up with the top of the scapula on one side and the humorous on the other. Well placed strikes will miss this muscle, but the odd errant swing of a flogger may catch it. This strong muscle protects the delicate ball and joint connection of the arm to the torso.

The real star of the show is the latissimus dorsi. It's the big slab of muscle that protects the back and is responsible for that well defined "V" shape that many muscular people have. This muscle covers the back of the ribs and also extends low enough on the back to protect most of the organs.

Of course, you do need to take the physical condition of your bottom into account. A person with less muscle mass and less body fat may not be able to handle heavier strikes, no matter how tough they are. Pain may not be the limiting factor, damage to the body can be. For this reason (among many) it is important to start light and work your way up to more intense play - see the chapter on warm-ups for more information. Achy for a few days after playing is fine, pain that lasts beyond that (depending on the intensity of play) is not a good sign. Listen to your body.

If shoulder blades are sticking out, this can also present a problem. Skin that is stretched tightly over bone is more likely to break or mark. There is also a good chance that the experience will be more painful for the bottom, perhaps in an unpleasant way.

If the protruding shoulder blades are due to the position, move your bottom to a more comfortable one. If it's due to low body mass, you may need to play a bit lighter or on a different part of the body.

The upper back is a favourite place for flogger strikes. Your aim must be perfected before trying to strike this part of the body as the chances for a misplaced blow are fairly high. An accidentally wrapped flogger can strike the face, arms, or chest. You also want to avoid hitting the spine during play. It's an important structure and should not be hit - your chiropractor will thank you!

Good, With a But...

These areas are good to play on but they do need some extra precautions (or they're a little outside of the traditional box). As long as everyone involved is aware of the risks and do what they need to mitigate them, these parts of the body can be a lot of fun for impact and pain play.

Chest/Breasts

This is a tricky one. Breast tissue is different than the skin, muscle and fat usually found in other parts of the body. All people have some degree of breast tissue unless it's been surgically excised. Yes, men have breast tissue too, just a lot less of it than women typically do. Estrogen spurs the development of breasts, so trans-women on hormones will develop breasts while women with estrogen deficiencies like Turner's syndrome may not.

All of this is relevant because of the way that breast tissue reacts to impact. When we hit breasts (or anywhere), we can cause tiny micro-bleeds deep in the tissue. In breast tissue, they can become calcified as they heal and over time, develop hard lumps. These calcifications can be mistaken for tumours when seen on a mammogram. If you engage in heavy breast impact and get regular mammograms, it is best to let the technician know about your extracurriculars - even if you claim "rugby injuries". In a worst-case scenario, calcifications could obscure an actual tumour from sight resulting in a false negative test.

Fat necrosis is another risk (it's a risk on any area of the body that has larger amounts of fat but is more common on the breasts) and another complication that could be mistaken for cancer. It can present as a lump found on self-screening, leading to unneeded stress. The lumps can change over time and are often removed surgically.

If a person has breast implants, very light or no impact play should be done on the breasts. There is a risk of rupturing the implant. It's best to talk to your surgeon about the types of activities you wish to engage in (again, rugby is a full-contact sport and a common scapegoat for kinksters).

Impact play on the breasts can be done with minimal risk. I prefer to keep play to surface oriented implements - stingy sensations - to help minimize the risks of damage to breast tissue. If you want to do thuddy or deep impact play on breasts, it's best to ease up on the intensity.

Arms

Yes, you read that correctly, I said arms. The reason it's in this category is that arms are not really a popular impact play zone. They do have the features we are looking for, large muscles and no organs or other structures close to the surface (for the most part). They are a smaller area and have joints on either side, so some precision is needed.

The top and outside of the upper arm and forearm are fairly tough and robust. The radial nerve can come close to the surface on the outside portion of the arm, a little higher than halfway between the elbow and shoulder. Avoid impact on this area, especially if the bottom complains of radiating pain (usually travelling towards the hand).

The inside of the arm is protected from the regular bumps and thumps of day to day life. This means it hasn't had a chance to toughen up yet, which means much more sensitivity for the sadistic top who chooses to exploit it. Use precision implements like canes or short paddles in this area. Have the bottom place their hands on their head to expose the underside of the arm. Make sure you aren't hitting the armpit or ditch (inside of the elbow) and you're good to go.

Stomach

The stomach is okay for some types of play and not great for others. Contrary to what you may have read in a popular fantasy/romance book that involves BDSM, flogging the stomach does not feel good for most people. There will always be one or two out there, but they are the exception, not the rule.

The stomach is also not the greatest place to do impact because you can really hurt someone. I know that boxers and MMA fighters get hit in the stomach all the time, but they do lots of things I wouldn't advise the average person to do. They're trained to take hits to the stomach. If you are too, have at it, but it's probably not going to be a lot of fun.

That said, there are other ways to cause pain that don't involve hitting. The use of other pain play techniques, like the liberal use of clothespins, can work well over the stomach. It is a more sensitive area, both physically and psychologically. You may need to experiment to find something that works for you.

Calves

Again, not the first place you would think of to hit a person. As usual, avoid the joints, in this case, the knee and the ankle. Keep the impact to the calf muscle, avoiding the lower part of the leg entirely.

Remember that places that aren't used to being hit will be more sensitive!

Areas You Should Avoid Until You Know More

There are a few areas of the body that you should be more careful about impact and pain play. I highly suggest taking an in-person class or at least a really good online workshop before attempting impact or pain play in these areas.

Genitals

I love torturing genitals. I need to get that out there before I continue.

There are some types of play that you can do on genitals that won't cause much damage. For instance, clothespins (a common example, it seems) can be applied without any real precautions and will cause a fair bit of pain going on and coming off. On the other hand, it really isn't a good idea to engage in something like heavy impact (busting) on genitals if you don't know what you're doing.

Briefly, vulvae are pretty tough. Impact isn't going to cause much damage, other than bruising, but I still don't suggest doing it without taking a class first. You know the rules - start light and slowly increase intensity if you are going to play.

Testicles can be pulled - slowly, don't yank on them. They can be squeezed. Be careful not to hit one or the other with too much force at once. Don't ever twist the scrotum, as this can cause a torsion. It's a very painful condition that requires immediate medical attention to save the testicle. Don't get into the more serious play without proper instruction.

Hands & Feet

I have a strange love of doing all the things I tell others not to do. I've taken classes, studied on my own and cautiously experimented over the years - which is exactly what I'm going to tell you to do too. I love bastinado (foot caning). I enjoy hand strapping as well. Both of these can cause damage to the delicate bones of the hands and feet if you aren't careful.

Any impact should be on the palms and soles. The tops of the hands and feet should never be hit. You must have impeccable aim with your chosen implement or else you can do a lot of damage. Take a class before proceeding.

Face

It really depends on what you want to do to the face. Slapping, while a popular activity, is often done wrong and can result in a lot of bad things happening. Orbital bones getting broken, eardrums ruptured, cauliflower ears from too hard, misplaced blows....

On the other hand, if you want to put some clamps on a tongue or prop open a mouth, you shouldn't have much trouble.

Impact on the head and face should be learned in person before attempting. It is important to support the head to protect the neck when striking. Again, your aim is so important, so make sure you won't miss.

No Way, No How

Which brings us to the areas that you should just avoid when it comes to impact and pain play. Now there will be some ways that you can cause pain safely to just about any area of the body. For instance, you wouldn't want to hit the back of the head with a paddle, but you can cause pain by grabbing a handful of hair. Take this into account when reading this section.

Head & Neck

The head and neck should not be used as a target for impact play (with limited exceptions for face slapping). I know boxers and football players get hit in the head all the time. Have you been reading the latest research about the damage repeated concussions can do to the brain?

The neck is obviously pretty delicate, at least when it comes to impact play. The back of it has all those bones that are protecting a big bundle of nerves and the front takes care of the transportation of blood and oxygen. Damage to the trachea can be deadly and it doesn't take that much force to damage it. If there is ever a time to err on the side of caution, this is it.

Joints

As I've already mentioned, it's best to avoid playing on joints. Impact for sure, but even other types of pain play can cause problems. Nerves, arteries, and veins are closer to the surface in the joints and are less protected than in other parts of the body. You don't want to damage them, so stay away.

Joints are also unstable when it comes to impact. They can easily be knocked out of alignment leading to pain and other problems. Also, it's just not going to feel good to get hit in the knee or elbow. Oh! Let's do some ankle play - said no one ever.

Don't forget that the hips are just big joints. You're fine to hit the buttocks as hard as pain tolerances and consent allows, but make sure you avoid the sides of the hips. They don't have the glutes protecting them in the same way.

Shins

If didn't include it, someone would try it. The shins are basically skin stretched over bone. It's not going to feel good to do impact there and it's much more likely for the skin to break. There is no fat or muscle cushion to absorb some of the impact, just the skin getting hit against bone. Don't do it.

Lower Back

While stories of light flogging sending people to the hospital with severe kidney damage are greatly exaggerated, there is a kernel of truth. The kidneys are mostly protected by the rib cage and the lats, but in some people, they do poke out the bottom. It would take some pretty intense impact to do damage, but it's certainly possible.

The lower back doesn't have a lot of fat or muscle to hit and there are organs under the skin, so really it's best to avoid. I will go back to the argument that it probably won't feel very good for the bottom either.

General Safety Issues

There are some general safety issues to be aware of when engaging in impact and pain play.

Repeated, heavy impact on one area of the body can cause tissues to harden over time. It's the natural reaction of the body - think about a callus built up in response to ill-fitting shoes. It takes years, even decades, but bottoms can develop what is known in the community as "leather butt". The skin is tougher, meaning they feel less, which leads to playing harder, which leads to more trauma and toughening of the skin. It's a vicious cycle and something that most masochists are destined to have happen.

To avoid leather butt, which can happen anywhere on the body, not just the butt, allow ample healing time between play scenes. It's the repeated trauma, especially trauma to unhealed tissue, that causes leather butt to form. If you allow for a long (weeks, a month) healing period before playing on that part of the body again, you may be able to stave off the worst of it.

Impact play can cause inflammation in the area of the body that has been hit. This can cause a number of problems. The first is nerve impingement. This is most commonly seen in the hips and buttocks, resulting in sciatica. It is not a common result of play and requires repeated, heavy play scenes in the same area. If you notice some radiating pain and haven't had any other injury, it may be inflammation from play. See your doctor, but don't rule out this possibility.

The other, much more rare, potential complication is a Marjolin's ulcer. These take years to form and repeated injury to the same area. This is a rare form of cancer that is best avoided by allowing an area to heal before engaging in impact play there again.

The good news here is that there are so many parts of the body that are fun for play. If you spank the buttocks today, tomorrow flog the upper back. Allow an area to heal before returning to it. You may even want to take a day or two away from the impact play - thank goodness there are so many other forms of play to explore!

You should keep in mind that bruises can take a few hours, even overnight, to show up. Every person will react differently to play. Those reactions won't always be the same either. Hydration levels, amount of sleep, age and so much more can change the way the body reacts to play. Be cautious in the beginning until you know how your partner (or your body) will generally react. If no marks are important to you, play a bit lighter.

As we age, our skin becomes thinner and fat deposits under the skin change. This means that older skin is more likely to bruise than younger skin. I know I've found that the changes in my skin have become more and more obvious as the years go on. Again, play a bit lighter until you know what to expect.

It's true that women tend to bruise easier than men. This is because women tend to have more subcutaneous fat and fatty areas of the body will bruise easier than muscled ones. Even a layer of fat over muscle means more bruising.

Hard implements and bony areas of the body do not mix. Skin that has little padding under it, so that it's laying on top of bone, is more likely to break than padded areas. Hard implements like paddles and canes make this effect worse.

Play Safe

There are a number of things you can do to ensure the safety of everyone during an impact and pain scene. Taking some simple precautions can prevent an awkward trip to the emergency room, so they're well worth it.

Make sure that the bottom is resting on a solid surface. Whether it's a St. Andrew's Cross or spanking bench at the local dungeon or laying face down on the bed, you want to make sure your bottom isn't going to fall if they get dizzy or lose consciousness. Don't risk an unstable surface. At best, it will distract your bottom so that they need to focus more on not falling rather than enjoying your scene.

Make sure that your bottom is positioned in such a way that you can hit the spot you want, without hitting the spots you don't want. For instance, if you're flogging the bottom's chest, have them tilt their head back. St. Andrew's crosses are great for this, as the space between the two arms allows the bottom to lean back without falling. Even if you don't have a cross, keeping their face out of the way of the falls is important.

You can also protect parts of the body by placing a toy, folded t-shirt or leather strap over them. As I suggested to protect the tailbone earlier, this trick can work with other parts of the body as well. Just don't let it become a substitute for practising your aim. If you are missing your mark frequently, go back to hitting a pillow until you improve.

If you have a bottom who moves a lot when hit, you may need to secure them using bondage. If you've told them to stay still and they just can't, you will need to make them. Hitting a moving target is much harder than a stationary one. Hitting a randomly moving target who is actively trying to avoid getting hit is a real challenge. You can easily end up with misplaced strikes that can cause harm.

The most important thing you can do to protect your bottom is to educate yourself and practice. There are so many resources available for those who want to learn. Practice takes time and patience. You need to be disciplined in order to become proficient in any skill. Keep hitting your pillows until it's perfect.

12 EXPLORING IMPACT & PAIN PLAY: CHECKLIST

Impact and pain play are broad categories that include simple activities like spanking with a bare hand to activities that take classes and many hours of practice, like using a single tail whip. Don't look over the checklist and expect to be able to do everything right away. I've marked the activities that are more suitable for beginners with a ✪ next to the activity. Skills that take a bit of leg work are marked with a 🕮 and activities that are the most difficult to do are indicated with a ⚐. Some activities can be a mixture of multiple levels, so I've included the relevant icons.

Don't be discouraged that you can't do everything on the list right now. Those activities are meant to give you inspiration and ideas for the future. Start with the simple activities and go from there. I have tried to include many easy to do activities that don't require any (or very inexpensive) specialized equipment. Hopefully, there will be at least 3 or so simple activities that you are interested in so that you can create an impact and pain play scene.

HOW TO USE THE CHECKLIST

You may find it easiest to photocopy this list or download it from my website at www.MsMorganThorne.com if you prefer to do it online or print it out yourself.

Both or all partners should fill out this checklist, to gauge interest in activities and so that they are aware of what the other(s) are interested in. If you have multiple partners, each pairing should fill out a checklist, as what you are willing to explore with one partner may be different than what you are willing to explore with another.

Make sure you indicate your experience, if any, with each activity. Again, this is the beginning of a conversation, not the whole thing. Don't be afraid to ask a person how they learned, whether they were a top or bottom for that activity, etc.

If an activity does not apply to you for whatever reason, simply ignore it or write in **N/A**.

Use a **T** or **B** to indicate that you would be interested in topping or bottoming for an activity. If you're interested in doing both, simply write both letters in.

Rating scale for the checklist.

Remember, if you haven't tried an activity, indicate your interest level in that activity. If you plan on having others involved directly in your play, indicate with an * which activities you would want to keep between you and your primary partner or the person you are filling this checklist out with.

- **NO** is a hard limit, something you are not interested in doing under any circumstances.
- **0** (zero) is a soft limit, something you aren't interested in doing, but may consider under specific circumstances and with specific negotiation.
- **1** (one) is something you aren't really interested in doing but will oblige if it's requested occasionally.
- **2** (two) is something that you're okay with doing but you don't really enjoy. You will do it if asked, to please your partner, or as a special reward.
- **3** (three) is something that you neither like nor dislike. You're up for it if your partner wants to, but it's not something you would miss if it didn't happen.
- **4** (four) is something you enjoy doing and wouldn't mind doing often.
- **5** (five) is something you really want to do, something you would like to do as often as possible.
- **?** is something you don't understand or are truly unsure about.

Explanations can be found online - but be careful what you search for, you may not like what you see!

Always remember that these checklists are not written in stone. You can change your checklist whenever you like. If you try something and it's not nearly as much fun as you thought it would be, change it's rating. If you didn't think you would like something but have warmed up to the idea, change it's rating. Don't forget to let your partner know about the change. These checklists are a great way to keep track of things and for spurring conversations, but most of us don't check them before each time we play. I recommend using pencil to fill out your checklist so that you can change it whenever you need.

There are blank spots at the end of each checklist. If there is something that fits this category that I haven't included, write it in! I've also done my best to keep the lists somewhat short, which means I've left out some of the more extreme activities. If you are interested in more extreme play, make sure you get educated on how to do it safely, including attending workshops and reading all you can on the subject.

Name: Date:

Impact & Pain Play Activity	Experience Y/N	Rating NO, 1-5, ?	Top or Bottom?
Abrasion ✪			
Bastinado (Foot Caning) 🕮			
Biting (No Marks) ✪			
Biting (Marks) ✪			
Caning (Body) 🕮			
Caning (Hands) 🕮			
Caning (Genitals) 🕮			
Clamps (Nipple) ✪			
Clamps (Genitals) ✪			
Clamps (Other, Lips, Tongue, etc) ✪			
DIY Implements ✪ 🕮 ⚐			
Electrical Play 🕮 ⚐			
Floggers (Leather, Suede, Fur) 🕮			
Floggers (Weights or Knots) ⚐			
Floggers (Rubber or Chain) ⚐			

Impact & Pain Play Activity	Experience Y/N	Rating NO, 1-5, ?	Top or Bottom?
Floggers (Genitals) 🕮			
Floggers (Breasts) 🕮			
Hair Pulling ✪			
Kicking ⚐			
Kicking (Ball or Cunt Busting) ⚐			
Kitchen Implements ✪			
Neon Wand 🕮			
Paddles (Wooden) ✪			
Paddles (Textured or Holes) 🕮			
Paddles (Unusual Size, Shape, Material) 🕮			
Paddles (Genitals) 🕮			
Paddles (Breasts) ✪			
Pain (Mild) ✪			
Pain (Moderate) ✪ 🕮			
Pain (Severe) 🕮 ⚐			
Riding Crops (Leather Tress) ✪			
Riding Crops (Rubber Tress) ✪			

Impact & Pain Play Activity	Experience Y/N	Rating NO, 1-5, ?	Top or Bottom?
Riding Crops (Other Tress) ✪			
Riding Crops (Breasts) ✪			
Riding Crops (Genitals) ✪			
Scratching (Fingernails) ✪			
Scratching (Metal "Claws") ✪			
Scratching (Other Implements) ✪			
Slapping (Body) ✪			
Slapping (Face) 🕮			
Slapping (Breasts) ✪			
Slapping (Genitals) ✪			
Spanking (Hands) ✪			
Spanking (Hair Brush) ✪			
Spanking (Over the Knee) ✪			
Straps (Leather) 🕮			
Straps (Rubber or Silicone) 🕮			
Straps (Hands) 🕮			
Straps (Breasts) 🕮			

Impact & Pain Play Activity	Experience Y/N	Rating NO, 1-5, ?	Top or Bottom?
Straps (Genitals) 🕮			
Tawse 🕮			
Tawse (Hands) 🕮			
Tawse (Breasts) 🕮			
Tawse (Genitals) 🕮			
TENS Units (Electrical) 🕮			
Violet Wand (Regular Electrodes) 🕮			
Violet Wand (Metal Electrodes) 🕮			
Violet Wand (Flogging) 🕮			
Violet Wand (Metal Objects) 🕮			
Violet Wand (Branding) ⚐			
Weights (Nipples) 🕮			
Weights (Genitals) 🕮			
Whips (Single Tail) ⚐			
Whips (Breasts) ⚐			
Whips (Genitals) ⚐			
Whips (Breaking Skin) ⚐			

Impact & Pain Play Activity	Experience Y/N	Rating NO, 1-5, ?	Top or Bottom?
Whips (Fear Play & Cracking) ⚐			
Wooden Spoon ✪			
Wrestling ✪ 🕮 ⚐			

13 EXPLORING IMPACT & PAIN PLAY: SCENE CREATION & IDEAS

Take a look at yours and your partner's lists. Are there activities that you are both interested in? Are there some areas where there are both interest and compatibility for topping and bottoming? Additionally, it is always wise to know what is off the table as well as what you're planning on doing. You don't want to have a moment of inspiration and do something your partner hates (you may want to review the chapters on Consent and Negotiation at this point).

For the sake of this exploration, we are going to say that anything rated 2/5 or lower is off limits for now. When you're playing in the future, you may want to negotiate the inclusion of some of those activities, but for now, this is more of a first taste - you don't want to have anything questionable in the mix.

IMPACT & PAIN PLAY SPECIFIC SAFETY CONCERNS

Obviously, impact and pain play can hold a lot of hazards. We are talking about striking people, often with objects that are unforgiving. If you want to try something, make sure you know what you're doing. I strongly suggest you attend classes and workshops on activities you wish to try. At the very least, watch instructional, non-porn videos and research as best you can. Resources for learning will be included in advanced learning .

I won't go into the safety concern for every item on the checklist, but I will talk about the ones that new folks are most likely to try. Always remember that BDSM is dangerous, so make sure you are confident that you and your partner know what you're getting into.

Nipple clamps are pretty easy to use. Pinch the nipple and place the clamp at the back of the nipple (or just behind for small nipples). It is important that clamps are not left on for too long. They cut off blood supply to the thing they are clamped onto. This goes for clamps on lips, labia, penis, scrotum, etc. 10-15 minutes is a good general rule to follow. A little longer won't be a big deal, but leave a clamp on for too much longer and you may run into trouble.

Another thing that people don't always realize with clamps is that they hurt more coming off than going on. The longer they are on, the more they will hurt when removed. This pain lasts for a while and is worse when the nipple (or whatever was clamped) is stimulated by touch. This can be used to your advantage if your partner is into the pain, or it can cause some to safe word. Make sure you don't overdo it.

Whips, floggers, canes, and other flexible implements can wrap around the body if not used properly. You must strike with the right part of the implement in order to avoid this. Wrapping is generally a sign of a person who does not know how to use the implement. It can cause serious damage to the bottom because the tips of the implements are moving much faster when they wrap. They can dig in and cause cuts, welts and other damage where it is not intended. For instance, if a person is flogging a bottom's back, the flogger could strike the shoulders or neck (which is off limits) and wrap around to the front of the body, hitting the throat, chest, or even the face. Once again, make sure you are educated in the use of an implement before you use it.

Hair pulling should be done by grabbing the hair as close to the roots as possible. It may seem sexy to grab hair and snap the head back, but be careful. You can injure the bottom's neck this way. Grab firmly and move the head without jerking.

Riding crops should always be used properly to avoid damage to both the bottom and the toy. Strike only with the tress, not the shaft. If you want something you can use as a cane, buy a cane. Crops are not designed to have force applied in that way on the shaft and can break, shattering and leaving shards in the bottom.

For clarity, you may want to organize those activities here;

Compatible activities rated 4/5 or higher:

Who will top? Who will bottom?

Compatible activities 3/5:

Who will top? Who will bottom?

Which activities are off the table (listed as 2/5 or lower)?

Planning Your Scene

Now, with any luck, you will have three or four (maybe even more) activities listed in the 4/5 and better category. If you don't, take a look at what is listed in the 3/5 category. Hopefully, you have enough activities to create a scene.

Ideally, you don't want to try to cram 1,000 things into a single scene. Stick to anywhere between three and five impact and pain play activities. These types of activities are relatively simple, most don't require any type of setup and many of the skills are easy to learn on your own.

One of the nice things about impact and pain play activities is that they do go well together. Once you have a bit of experience under your belt, you will be able to incorporate more activities into your play scenes. For now, though, let's just stick to the three to five activities, so you don't feel overwhelmed.

Don't feel like you have to go on forever when you're first exploring. Sometimes 15 or 30 minutes is enough to do what you want to do and leave you wanting a bit more. A common way that people trip themselves up is thinking that they have to create huge, elaborate, and long play scenes that will take up a whole night. They often spend more time watching the clock rather than just letting things flow naturally.

Set a shorter time limit to your activities, but let it be flexible. If things are going well and you play for an extra 10 minutes, great! If it's just not working and you decide to wrap up one activity sooner, so you can move on to something more enjoyable, that's perfectly okay! Would you rather continue something that neither of you is enjoying because you will be 5 minutes short in your scene? Sounds pretty silly, doesn't it? If something isn't working, move on to the next thing and try not to sweat it. You can always revisit later.

Let's create an example couple, Jamie and Taylor. They will walk us through each area of exploration and serve as an example of how you can explore BDSM. Please note I've tried to choose gender-neutral names and will be using they/their as pronouns for this fictitious couple.

Jamie & Taylor's Checklist & Negotiation

Both Jamie and Taylor have filled out the Impact and Pain Play Checklist. They have listed their mutual 4/5 and above activities. They are nipple clamps, hand spanking, wooden spoons, and paddles.

They want to pick one more activity to round out the scene, so they turn to their list of 3/5s. Jamie has listed biting (no marks) as a 3/5. Taylor has rated it 5/5.

After a bit of discussion, Jamie agrees that the inclusion of biting without marks would be a nice addition to the scene. It's not Jamie's favourite thing, but knowing that Taylor really likes it makes it more appealing.

They've also found that Jamie is more interested in topping for activities, while Taylor is interested in bottoming.

Jamie and Taylor already have a romantic and sexual relationship. They agree that this scene will be like foreplay, include some sexual touching and kissing, ending with a transition to sex. They've also agreed that since this is their first foray into the world of BDSM, they will be using an opt-in style of negotiation, at least until the end of the kink part of the scene. They have well established sexual chemistry and don't feel the need to negotiate that portion of the scene.

Even though they know each other well, they decide to go over any hard limits and health concerns. Jamie has asthma and makes sure that Taylor knows where the inhaler is. Taylor has choking as a hard limit and reminds Jamie of this.

They agree to use the stoplight system of safe words. Jamie will check in with Taylor by asking "what's your colour?" or by simply saying "You like that, don't you?" and other similar things.

They will be playing at Jamie's home, where they won't be disturbed. They expect that the BDSM portion of their scene will take about half an hour.

Neither of them are sure if they will need aftercare, so they agree to their usual routine of cuddling after sex followed by a cup of tea and a light snack. They also agree that if either of them needs something more, they will speak up and ask for it (while also paying attention to the other, in case they need comfort but are unable to ask for it).

Jamie & Taylor's Scene

Taylor arrives at Jamie's house. Both are nervous, knowing what they have planned for the evening. Taylor has brought a paddle that they found at a sex shop that sells BDSM toys created by local artisans. They couldn't find any nipple clamps that they both liked, so they will be using bamboo clothespins from the dollar store. While they were there, they also bought a wooden spoon to go in the kink chest, thinking it might be weird to use an actual cooking utensil.

They eat a nice dinner and start to relax a bit. After dinner, they have a soda and talk about how excited they are to try this BDSM scene together. They go over the details again, making sure they have everything they need. Once that is done, they head to the bedroom to get started.

When they arrive, it feels awkward. They both burst out laughing, they haven't been this nervous around each other since their first date! The laughter helps a bit, lightening the mood. Still laughing, Jamie pulls Taylor across their lap.

Jamie gives a light, playful smack on Taylor's ass. They both giggle and Jamie does it again, a bit harder this time. Taylor lets out a "mmmm...." and wiggles their ass a little at Jamie. Jamie starts trying to pull down Taylor's pants, Taylor eagerly helps.

They both strip down nude, feeling more comfortable that way. They spend some time kissing and touching each others bodies. Jamie starts mixing some light bites in with the kisses all over Taylor's body, while also grabbing at Taylor's ass.

This time, Taylor bends over the bed, looking over their shoulder at Jamie seductively. Jamie takes the hint and begins lightly spanking Taylor. Jamie is sure to move the swats around, never landing a blow in the same spot twice. The swats get progressively harder as the two get more and more aroused.

Jamie looks over to the bedside table and sees the spoon, paddle and clothespins. Reaching over and grabbing the clothespins for Taylor's nipples. Once affixed, Jamie returns to spanking. Taylor is moved forward slightly as each blow lands, jiggling the clothespins a bit and sending waves of sensation through Taylor's body.

Jamie now reaches for the paddle. It is slightly flexible and made of leather. They know from trying it out in the store that it is slightly stingy but delivers a good thud on harder strikes. Jamie uses it lightly at first, slowly building the intensity, in the same manner as the hand spanking.

Taylor is moaning loudly now and starting to have a hard time standing. They move to the middle of the bed, Taylor trying to lay down and promptly remembering the clothespins. Jamie reaches around and slowly removes the first one. As the blood rushes back into the nipple, Taylor is hit with a wave of intense sensation that is part pain and part pleasure. Jamie asks "are you ready for the next one" and removes it when Taylor nods.

Taylor collapses on the bed with Jamie now returning to hand spanking, the wooden spoon totally forgotten. Straddling Taylor's legs, Jamie leans down and begins to kiss Taylor's back while also reaching around and tweaking a nipple every now and then. Taylor turns around for a kiss and the couple transition into the sexual part of the scene.

What Can We Learn?

As you can see from our above example, you don't have to do everything on your list if it doesn't fit, you change your mind, or just forget. Sometimes you will get so wrapped up in the fun that you totally forget something you planned on doing. Don't sweat it, it happens to all of us from time to time.

Nervousness and awkwardness at the beginning are also completely normal. Don't be afraid to laugh. Laugh at yourselves, at the situation, at how nervous you are. Laughter is fun and can be sexy. How many times have you been enjoying a good laugh with a lover that has turned into something sexual? Use the positive energy between you to transition into the scene if it works for you.

Despite agreeing to check in verbally, Jamie only did so once. Taylor's reactions and actions told the story so words weren't needed throughout much of the scene. Wiggling their ass is a delicious way that many bottoms have of saying "come get me". Bending over with an inviting look says the same thing. We can make these interpretations of the body language because we know that these two had negotiated and agreed to engage in this type of play and because they have a long history together. If you're ever unsure or you don't know the person well, it's best to get verbal confirmation.

The other thing I wanted to point out here is that Taylor, the bottom in this scenario, is quite eager. While Jamie wasn't exactly hesitant, it can happen that tops get cold feet when it comes time to play.

Overcoming Childhood Programming

Some tops find it difficult to overcome the programming that we all get as children that it's bad to hit people. It's bad to cause pain to people, especially people we like or love. This is even more pronounced in male tops with female bottoms who have been told that they should never hit women. The messaging, intended to prevent domestic violence, is important to impart to children (preferably the nobody should ever hit anyone else without consent type) but can backfire for those into BDSM.

Tops can feel like monsters, assholes, evil, or any number of other negative things. My best advice is to take things slow. Bottoms should also be very clear in their consent and display how much they are enjoying the activity.

Even if you're someone who wants to try resistance play, if you are or are playing with a top who has trouble separating BDSM hitting from their childhood programming, it should be put to the back burner for a time. As the top gains confidence and is able to get past any feelings of guilt, the idea can be introduced slowly. Imagine, a person who is feeling like a monster already, with a partner who is yelling "no stop!" as they play. It can be enough for some tops to walk away entirely.

I have had luck helping tops through this hesitation by pointing out that their partner is asking for this activity. Not in a "look at that short skirt, she's totally asking for it" sort of way, but in an "I want you to smack my ass" kind of way. Reminding the nervous top of that hopefully enthusiastic consent, that the bottom has a safe word to stop things if needed, and seeing the bottom's enjoyment of the pain can get many tops past this roadblock.

Aftercare is important for many people. In this case, the top may need reassurance from the bottom in the form of cuddling, thanking them for a good time, and talking about the experience. If a top can hear and see how much a bottom is enjoying things, it can help them get past the programming and embrace their chosen role. Some turn out to be quite the sadists.

Some tops never get past this programming or they can only go so far before the guilt kicks in. That's totally okay. Tops are allowed limits too. It doesn't make them any less, it doesn't mean they are a bad top and it has nothing to do with dominance (as some people believe). If a top can enjoy spanking but not severe beatings that leave huge bruises and breaks skin, that is fine. They may find they enjoy being a more sensual top, engaging in sensation play rather than pain play. They may need to find a bottom who enjoys spanking and play that doesn't leave big bruises.

Trust me, while you may see the more severe stuff at parties or in pictures, most people don't play to that extreme regularly. There are people who enjoy all sorts of play, some fall into the "mild" camp and others fall into the "extreme" camp. Most are somewhere in between.

14 EXPLORING IMPACT & PAIN PLAY: SCENE REVIEW

You and your partner may want to shift into aftercare mode when you're done a scene, or you may find that you don't need it. You're not going to really know until you try a few scenes and see how you feel afterwards.

For many people, BDSM play will act as foreplay with sex as the main event. In that case, the sex itself can be viewed as aftercare. You may consider the typical cuddling after sex to be aftercare and not need anything further.

Some people don't have a sexual relationship or don't mix sex and BDSM. For them, they may still want to cuddle after play. Or they may have something totally different in mind. I've had partners who wanted to have a shower when we finished playing because they found it grounded them. Others have wanted to sit with me and chat about the weather, politics, or just anything. The conversation helped connect us and bring them back to reality. Still, others have just wanted to spend a bit of time sitting quietly and taking in the sensations and feelings that play brought up.

How ever you want to do aftercare is right for you. For more information about aftercare, please refer to the chapter on aftercare .

Impact & Pain Play Specific Aftercare

When we are playing in such physical ways, there are things we should do to take care of our partners when we are done. It's unethical to leave a partner who may be injured or in some sort of distress to their own devices (and that goes for any sort of play).

Bottoms should be checked for any cuts, bruising, inflammation, or bleeding. Apply first aid as needed. If there are signs of bruising, such as tiny red spots on the skin, and bruising is not desired, applying an ice pack can help prevent some of the bruising.

Some people find that arnica gel or lotions containing arnica can help prevent bruising. There is no scientific information on this subject (at the time of printing), but it won't do any harm if you choose to try it. Other people find that applying a good lotion or body butter, especially containing ingredients such as vitamin E, coconut oils, jojoba oils, or shea butter can help keep skin soft and supple. While it's unclear if this can prevent things like leather butt, those ingredients are well known for being good for the skin in general.

On that note, tops may also find that they have some swelling in hands if they have been spanking hard or sore muscles from swinging a flogger. Again, applying ice to swollen hands can help bring down swelling. The use of creams that warm up or heating pads can help with sore muscles. There has been more than once that I had a pretty sore arm and shoulder after a particularly intense and drawn out scene - I love my heating pad in those situations.

Both partners may need some emotional support after the scene. We covered some issues that the top may have in the previous chapter. Bottoms can also feel guilty, for the things they desire or the things they allowed the top to do to them. They should be reassured that desires for BDSM are not unhealthy as long as they are approached in a consensual manner. The guilt that society places on us for our desires can be hard to overcome, for people on both sides of the slash. Supportive partners, whether romantic, platonic or otherwise are essential to overcoming guilt around BDSM desires.

This is one of many reasons that I encourage people to seek out their local community. Seeing healthy, well-adjusted people engaging in kink in a consensual and healthy manner can help erase some of the negative programmings that our sex-negative and kink-negative society has left us with (thankfully, it does seem like things are changing for the better).

Finally, it is always wise to look over your toys and clean them at the end of a scene. For me, this is my time to centre myself and process what happened in the scene. I clean each toy as well as our dungeon furniture carefully, inspecting each one for signs of imperfection or damage that needs attention. If something is broken or damaged during the scene, I put it aside to see if it can be fixed later. If not, it gets thrown out and I make a mental note to pick up another.

To clean the toys and furniture, I usually use antibacterial wipes, giving each one a good rub down. If something has come in contact with blood, I need to evaluate if it's cleanable. If it's a single-use item, it gets disposed of in the proper manner (sharps in the sharps bin, soiled gauze in a double garbage bag). If it's a toy made of non-porous material, it gets sprayed down with hospital grade disinfectant according to the instructions. If it can be sterilized in an autoclave, it will be. I own an autoclave, something most people do not. You may achieve a similar temporary sterility by baking the item in the oven at low temperatures for a few hours. The item will be safe to touch and use but will no longer be sterile when you remove it from the oven (so it's a good tactic for toys that don't need to be sterile during use, but not a solution for things like sounds that need to be sterile when inserted).

If an item has come into contact with blood and is a porous material - a rattan cane, for example - I will clean it with the hospital grade disinfectant and gift it to the bottom. It will only be used on them from that point onward, regardless of who holds onto the item. You can not properly sterilize porous materials, so it is unsafe to use on other people.

I prefer to clean my own toys, because I'm very particular about it and, as I said, it has become my time to reflect on the scene. Some people will have the bottom clean up the toys and area after a scene. Others will do it together. How you approach this is entirely up to you.

Reviewing the Scene

Part of this exploration is figuring out what you enjoy and what is better left to fantasy. It is important that you sit down after your scene - shortly after or a few days after, it's up to you - and talk about it.

If you want a few days to process how you're feeling about the scene, that's fine. It is something you should communicate to your partner, so they don't become worried about why you aren't talking about it (the mind can lead to all sorts of scary places when it's worried). You may also want to keep a journal of your feelings or at least write down a few notes so that you don't forget anything important when it is time to talk.

You will need to figure out what exactly you need to cover in this post scene discussion, but I have provided some example questions that you should both answer. Compare your answers and talk about why they are the same or different. Did one person have a drastically different interpretation of part of the scene? Why do you think that happened?

It can be difficult to hear that your partner was hurt by a part of the scene that you thought went well or enjoyed. It can feel like criticisms or an attack on the top. That is the last thing that this should become. You're a team, and in order to ensure that both people are enjoying things, you will need to talk about both the good and the bad. Communication about these things can be hard, but it's such an important skill. This is especially true if you plan on trying edge play, pushing boundaries, or other more dangerous play in the future.

What parts of the scene did you enjoy? What was your favourite? Why?

How did those parts of the scene make you feel? Why do you think that is?

Were those parts things you had highly rated? Were there any pleasant surprises (things you weren't sure about but really enjoyed)?

Was there a part of the scene that you didn't enjoy?

Was it something you thought you would enjoy? Why do you think that it wasn't as good as you thought it would be?

How would you rate the intensity of the scene? Too low? Just right? Too much?

Would you be interested in trying that activity again or would you prefer to leave it for a while (or permanently)?

Was there anything that you felt you needed that you didn't get in the scene?

How do you think the scene went overall?

Did you find that the aftercare was sufficient? Did you drop?

Name one thing you would change for next time and one thing you would like to keep the same.

Feel free to add any questions that you think are important. Remember that BDSM isn't just a physical experience, it's a mental and emotional one too. Make sure you address all of these aspects when you have your scene review. Even though it may be hard, it is really important, to be honest with your partner, otherwise, they may end up doing things you don't enjoy inadvertently.

15 EXPLORING SENSATION PLAY: CHECKLIST

Sensation play tends to be more sexual but it doesn't have to be. It can be good, clean fun without a sensual or sexual component. It's up to you how you approach it.

Most of the items on this list are easy for beginners to pick up, these are marked with ✪. Some may require some research or a special purchase, marked with 🕮. Finally, there is the odd activity that does require in person instruction or can be greatly enhanced by it, indicated with ⚐.

This is probably the easiest subsection of BDSM to explore and can be a lot of fun on it's own or incorporated into a more involved scene. Sensation play is very versatile, it can be used as a reward and as funishment (think too much of a good thing). Have fun exploring!

How to Use this Checklist

You may find it easiest to photocopy this list or download it from my website at www.MsMorganThorne.com if you prefer to do it online or print it out yourself. Of course, you're more than welcome to fill out this one right here in the book if you want to keep things all in one place.

Both or all partners should fill out this checklist, to gauge interest in activities and so that they are aware of what the other(s) are interested in. If you have multiple partners, each pairing should fill out a checklist, as what you are willing to explore with one partner may be different than what you are willing to explore with another.

Make sure you indicate your experience, if any, with each activity. Again, this is the beginning of a conversation, not the whole thing. Don't be afraid to ask a person how they learned, whether they were a top or bottom for that activity, etc.

If an activity does not apply to you for whatever reason, simply ignore it or write in **N/A**.

Use a **T** or **B** to indicate that you would be interested in topping or bottoming for an activity. If you're interested in doing both, simply write both letters in.

Rating scale for the checklist.

Remember, if you haven't tried an activity, indicate your interest level in that activity. If you plan on having others involved directly in your play, indicate with an * which activities you would want to keep between you and your primary partner or the person you are filling this checklist out with.

- **NO** is a hard limit, something you are not interested in doing under any circumstances.
- **0** (zero) is a soft limit, something you aren't interested in doing, but may consider under specific circumstances and with specific negotiation.
- 1 (one) is something you aren't really interested in doing but will oblige if it's requested occasionally.
- **2** (two) is something that you're okay with doing but you don't really enjoy. You will do it if asked, to please your partner, or as a special reward.
- **3** (three) is something that you neither like nor dislike. You're up for it if your partner wants to, but it's not something you would miss if it didn't happen.
- **4** (four) is something you enjoy doing and wouldn't mind doing often.
- **5** (five) is something you really want to do, something you would like to do as often as possible.
- **?** is something you don't understand or are truly unsure about.

Explanations can be found online - but be careful what you search for, you may not like what you see!

Always remember that these checklists are not written in stone. You can change your checklist whenever you like. If you try something and it's not nearly as much fun as you thought it would be, change it's rating. If you didn't think you would like something but have warmed up to the idea, change it's rating. Don't forge to let your partner know about the change. These checklists are a great way to keep track of things and for spurring conversations, but most of us don't check them before each time we play. I recommend using pencil to fill out your checklist so that you can change it whenever you need.

There are blank spots at the end of each checklist. If there is something that fits this category that I haven't included, write it in! I've also done my best to keep the lists somewhat short, which means I've left out some of the more extreme activities. If you are interested in more extreme play, make sure you get educated on how to do it safely, including attending workshops and reading all you can on the subject.

Name: Date:

Sensation Play Activity	Experience Y/N	Rating NO, 1-5, ?	Top or Bottom
Abrasion ✪			
Caressing ✪			
Chemical Play 🕮 ⚐			
Chemical Play (Cooling Gels) 🕮			
Chemical Play (Hot Oil) 🕮			
Chemical Play (Icy Hot) 🕮			
Chemical Play (Numbing Creams) 🕮			
Chemical Play (Warming & Tingling Creams) 🕮			
Clothespins ✪			
Cupping (Suction) 🕮			
Cupping (Fire) 🕮 ⚐			
Electrical Play (Neon Wand) 🕮			
Electrical Play (TENS) 🕮			

Sensation Play Activity	Experience Y/N	Rating NO, 1-5, ?	Top or Bottom
Electrical Play (Violet Wand) 🕮 ⚐			
Electrical Play (Other) 🕮 ⚐			
Figging 🕮			
Fire Play ⚐			
Gas Masks ✪ 🕮 ⚐			
Hair Pulling ✪			
Hair Brushing ✪			
Ice Cubes ✪			
Latex/Rubber Clothing ✪ 🕮			
Leather Clothing ✪ 🕮			
Licking (Non-sexual) ✪			
Massage ✪			
Massage (Hot Oil) ✪			
Pumping (Pussy) 🕮			
Pumping (Clit) 🕮			
Pumping (Cock) 🕮			
Pumping (Nipples) 🕮			

Sensation Play Activity	Experience Y/N	Rating NO, 1-5, ?	Top or Bottom
Pumping (Other) 🕮			
Scratching (Fingernails) ✪			
Scratching (Metal Claws) ✪ 🕮			
Scratching (Other Implements) ✪			
Sensory Deprivation (Blindfold) ✪			
Sensory Deprivation (Sound) ✪			
Sensory Deprivation (Hoods) 🕮			
Sensory Deprivation (Body Bags) 🕮			
Sensory Deprivation (Other) 🕮			
Tickling ✪			
Tickling (Feet) ✪			
Tickling (Under Arms) ✪			
Tickle Torture ✪			
Vacuum Bed 🕮 ⚐			
Vibrators on Genitals ✪			
Vibrators Elsewhere ✪			
Wax Play 🕮			

Sensation Play Activity	Experience Y/N	Rating NO, 1-5, ?	Top or Bottom
Weights (Genital) 🕮			
Weights (Nipple) 🕮			
Weights (Other) 🕮			

16 EXPLORING SENSATION PLAY: SCENE CREATION AND IDEAS

Sensation play is often more sensual in nature, focusing on pleasure rather than pain. Of course, a good top understands that there can be too much of a good thing. Overloading the senses can ruin a scene or it can be a deliberate method to “torture” a bottom. Know and discuss your intentions beforehand (as always) and have a safe word in place.

Sensation play can easily cross the line over into sensual and sexual play. Make sure you negotiate clear boundaries around these activities. Do not assume that because you have an established sexual relationship that your partner wants to include sex in the scene. It’s very easy to simply ask and know for sure. BDSM doesn’t do well with assumptions.

A Note on Wax Play

I do want to point out that wax play may seem very straightforward. Sadly, I hear all too often from people who are hesitant or downright terrified of wax play because it’s so painful. This confused me in the beginning because my experience of way play is that it’s a mild, enjoyable sensation play activity.

With further investigation, I found that they were inexperienced and engaging with others who were similarly inexperienced. They used candles bought from a discount or dollar store. They use scented candles. They used glitter candles. Basically, they did all the things you’re not supposed to do!

It’s no wonder that they found wax play to be an awful experience. I’m surprised that more of these people didn’t have scars to show. Wax play is a pretty simple activity, but you need to know what the right materials are.

You should only ever use candles that are designed for wax play. If you are experienced and understand the melting points of various types of wax, you can make your own candles or occasionally find some in regular stores (but those usually don't list ingredients and have various additives that change the temperature of the wax).

Personally, I only use candles that are specifically designed for use on people. I prefer soy candles, as I find the soy/paraffin combination is sometimes too soft. The ones I buy are dyed with special dyes that don't alter the temperature of the wax (red and black are a few degrees hotter, but the vendor is able to tell me that up front).

Long story short: don't do wax play with discount candles or ones bought from regular stores. They are too hot and will burn your bottom. ONLY use candles which are designed for wax play.

Sensation Play Specific Safety Concerns

If you choose to engage in electrical play, you should always get educated on it first. Engaging in electro play with people who have heart conditions, pacemakers, electronic implants (insulin or pain pumps), epilepsy, and various other medical conditions is extremely dangerous. Do not engage without consulting a cardiologist or other appropriate doctor first.

Sensory deprivation can cause some people to panic. It's best to progress slowly with sensory deprivation, by only restricting one sense at a time, to begin with. You can add other senses as you both feel more comfortable, but don't add bondage yet. When you feel the time is right, slowly introduce bondage, restraining feet only or one hand, one foot at first, then moving to more and more strict bondage. If at any point the bottom feels panic rising up, they should indicate their safe word or signal. Their senses should be returned at the first instance of safe signalling, starting with the blindfold. Many people will feel more calm if they can see. It should always be the first thing you remove if you feel the bottom is in distress.

Gas masks can be used to restrict breathing. If you are using them in this way, be sure to have a safe signal in place. Also, know that it is very dangerous to restrict breathing to the point of unconsciousness. A book for beginner play is not the place to elaborate on the dangers of restricting breathing (which is advanced edge play at best), More on this in the Exploring Taboo and Edge Play.

Planning Your Scene

For each type of play, you will follow the same basic structure that we discussed in Impact & Pain Play Scene Creation & Ideas (page 86).

Once again, you will want to agree on three to five activities that you want to try. Make sure you select from the beginner activities unless you've had the chance to learn some of the others (or you have the specialized equipment for them).

List your activities that rate 4/5 or higher, next are the activities that are 3/5. Anything which scored 2/5 or lower should be off-limits for the time being. When you're first exploring, it's best to stick to things that both partners are really into. Pushing limits or trying things you're unsure about can come later, once you have some good experiences under your belt.

Compatible activities rated 4/5 or higher:

Who will top? Who will bottom?

Compatible activities 3/5:

Who will top? Who will bottom?

Which activities are off the table (listed as 2/5 or lower)?

Jamie & Taylor's Exploration

Jamie and Taylor are at it again. Now they want to explore sensation play. They have listed abrasion, clothespins, ice cubes, blindfolds, and tickling as 4/5 activities. They decide that they have already tried clothespins, so they would rather explore something different this time. They turn to their 3/5 list and find that Jamie has put wax play on that list. They don't have proper candles, so they agree to use some hot massage oil they got in a sample pack from the sex store.

With the activities decided, they choose that Jamie will again be topping for most of the scene. Taylor thinks it might be fun to try some things on Jamie too, so they agree that they will switch for the ice cubes and hot oil, taking turns.

Their other negotiation is similar to their impact scene. They expect that this scene will again lead to sex and that some sexual touching and kissing is okay during the scene. They go over their hard limits and health concerns, reminding each other of this important information. The scene will again happen at Jamie's and last for around half an hour. Safe words are the same and since they aren't using a gag, they don't feel the need for a safe signal.

They assemble the items they need in the bedroom. This includes a glass of ice, the hot oil (it's a candle that you light, which melts into massage oil), a variety of items for abrasion play including a plastic dish scrubber, some wooden skewers, and a plastic back scratcher. Jamie will use fingernails as well. They almost forgot a lighter for the candle but remembered at the last minute.

Play Time

This time, things aren't as awkward when they make their way to the bedroom. This scene feels more like elaborate sex than BDSM for them, something they are a bit more comfortable with. Jamie has Taylor strip and lay down face up on the bed. Jamie stays dressed.

Jamie places the blindfold on Taylor and lights the massage oil candle. Jamie isn't quite sure where to start, as there are so many choices to make. Jamie decides to start with the plastic back scratcher. Taylor doesn't really react to it. Jamie tries pressing a bit harder without any reaction.

Jamie abandons that toy and begins to gently rub hands over Taylor. Taylor jumps and giggles every time Jamie's hands go over their belly. Jamie decides to alternate tickling Taylor with lightly drawing the skewer over their skin. This gets the proper reaction; Taylor is writhing and giggling, unsure of what's coming next. Jamie adds the plastic scrubber as well, which adds to the tickling sensation.

After playing around with those toys for a while, Jamie really starts tickling Taylor. It's not long before Taylor calls out yellow, gasping for breath. Jamie figures it's time to move on anyway and gets Taylor to turn over.

The massage oil candle has had lots of time to melt and warm up. Jamie pours a small amount on Taylor's back and starts rubbing. Jamie also grabs an ice cube and runs it down Taylor's spine. The contrast between the two sensations has Taylor moaning. Jamie decides that since they agreed to sexual play, to drip some of the massage oil on Taylor's butt cheeks and rub it down towards Taylor's genitals.

Jamie continues playing with the contrast of the hot oil and cold ice all over Taylor's body. Eventually, Taylor is overcome with passion and removes the blindfold. They hadn't really talked about how they would indicate it was time to switch, so Taylor gently pushes Jamie towards the bed, pulling off pants as they lay down. Once Jamie is free of clothing, Taylor turns the tables, using the hot oil and ice on Jamie. Of course, this only lasts for a short while before the two transition into sexual activity.

What Can We Learn?

In this scene, we see a few different things from the first one. The first is that it is very easy to forget small parts of your toys when preparing for a scene. I can't tell you how many times I've forgotten a lighter or some other small thing for a scene. As a result, I have a number of lighters around my dungeon and I always keep one with the wax play candles and fire cups.

Make sure you go over each item and have what you need to make it work. Have condoms for insertables (if you plan on using condoms for those), have lighters for candles. It's also a good idea to have a towel if you're playing with ice because it makes a bit of a mess when it melts. Use enough and you will have a rather large wet spot to deal with.

The first "toy" that Jamie tried didn't work out. It didn't get the reaction they wanted or any reaction at all. It's okay. Some things won't work out the way you want. Just put them aside and move on to the next thing. Just make sure that your bottom isn't the stoic type! Stoic bottoms can be hard to read because they don't have much of a reaction to things. This is where knowing your partner and their reactions come in handy. If you're in doubt, check in and ask.

In this scenario, Taylor called yellow. This generally means that a bottom is close to their limit and can't take much more of this activity (of course, you can negotiate a different meaning if you choose). Tickling is one of those activities that will make almost any bottom safe word. I've had bottoms who you could beat bloody and they would ask for more. Tickling would always result in a "RED!!"

Jamie chose to move to a different activity when yellow was called. You can try a few different things in this situation, depending on what you've negotiated. You can say "just a few more" continuing for a short time before moving on. You can keep going until you get a red/safe word. You can move on immediately. You can always return to that activity once the person has had a chance to recover a bit, or you may want to leave it alone for the rest of that scene.

Since the two hadn't discussed how they would indicate time to switch, it was up in the air. In this case, they were both agreeable to it. If you choose to switch during a scene, you may want to set a specific time when that will happen (after I do this, you take over). You may want to go back and forth, trading off after each activity or randomly. Some switches like to "fight" for control. Others will switch at some point and not switch back. Basically, it's totally up to you and your partner, there is no wrong way to switch.

17 EXPLORING SENSATION PLAY: AFTERCARE AND SCENE REVIEW

Don't fall into the trap of thinking that because no one was causing pain during a scene that some people may not need aftercare. Sensation scenes can be just as intense, albeit in a different way than impact or pain focused scenes.

As usual, some people will need aftercare and others will not. When you're first exploring, it may be wise to err on the side of caution and do some form of aftercare. If you find later that you don't need it, you're fine to drop it. If you do need aftercare or need different things, you can adjust as needed.

Sensation Play Specific Aftercare

There are a few things that are specific to sensation play activities that you may want to look out for.

If you have explored chemical play in the form of warming creams and similar, these can be difficult to neutralize. It is always wise to learn what you will need to use to neutralize the specific thing that you've used during play, as each can be different.

Tiger Balm is a commonly used chemical, it can be neutralized with some olive oil (other oils work as well) on a cotton ball followed by dish soap and water. Make sure you wipe off any excess before applying oil. This works for Bengay, Icy Hot, as well as various muscle and arthritis creams.

These chemicals can become very intense very quickly. I learned the hard way, through mistaking a warming muscle cream for a different medicated lotion that placing warming chemicals over large parts of the body can create problems with body temperature regulation. I ended up shivering in a hot shower in the middle of the summer because of that mistake (and it wasn't even BDSM related, so I didn't get to have any fun).

The common ingredient in the above-listed ointments is Methyl Salicylate. Always look at the label before play so that you can have a way to neutralize it on hand - you don't want to go running to the kitchen looking for the olive oil when your partner has burning genitals!

For creams that contain capsaicin (or if you just applied the hot peppers directly), use a cotton ball soaked in vinegar, apple cider vinegar, or milk. All three will work to ease the burn. Running the area under cool water afterwards will also help ease the pain.

If you've played with cupping, you may have hard, raised circles on your skin. There isn't much that can be done for the bruising. The hardness, caused by lymph coming to the surface of the skin, can be helped with some light massage. It will also go away on its own over time (a few hours, usually).

If you've done electrical play, the bottom should be checked for burns. This is especially true if you were using metal electrodes on a violet wand. Burns are rare but can happen if you don't move the electrode enough.

Fire play dries out the skin, so some sort of moisturizing lotion should be included in the aftercare. Check for burns, blisters and broken skin first, applying first aid as needed.

Clean up for wax play or any play involving oils is much easier if you use a drop cloth first. Most BDSM wax will melt off in a hot shower, but you will want to remove as much as possible first so that you don't clog up your pipes. The skin should be checked for burns and lotion applied when you're done. Most BDSM candles will have some amount of soy oil in them, which helps protect the skin, but a nice body rub with lotion is generally enjoyable.

Reviewing the Scene

Hopefully, your scene went well. Most people will feel more comfortable with sensation play activities than with impact or pain play activities. This can be good, they will have more confidence and perhaps already have some degree of knowledge regarding the activity. On the other hand, some people view sensation play as more tame or safe, and they can get careless during play.

It can be hard if you need to hold your partner accountable for a cavalier attitude towards safety, but it's better to do it now, rather than when doing edge play later on. Even if you don't ever intend on doing edge play, do you really want a partner who has a cavalier attitude towards safety in any context?

Sensation play can also be very different for different people. A sensation that is pleasurable to one can be uncomfortable or even painful for another. This is the time to bring up any issues, as well as talking about the good stuff.

What parts of the scene did you enjoy? What was your favourite? Why?

How did those parts of the scene make you feel? Why do you think that is?

Were those parts things you had highly rated? Were there any pleasant surprises (things you weren't sure about but really enjoyed)?

Was there a part of the scene that you didn't enjoy?

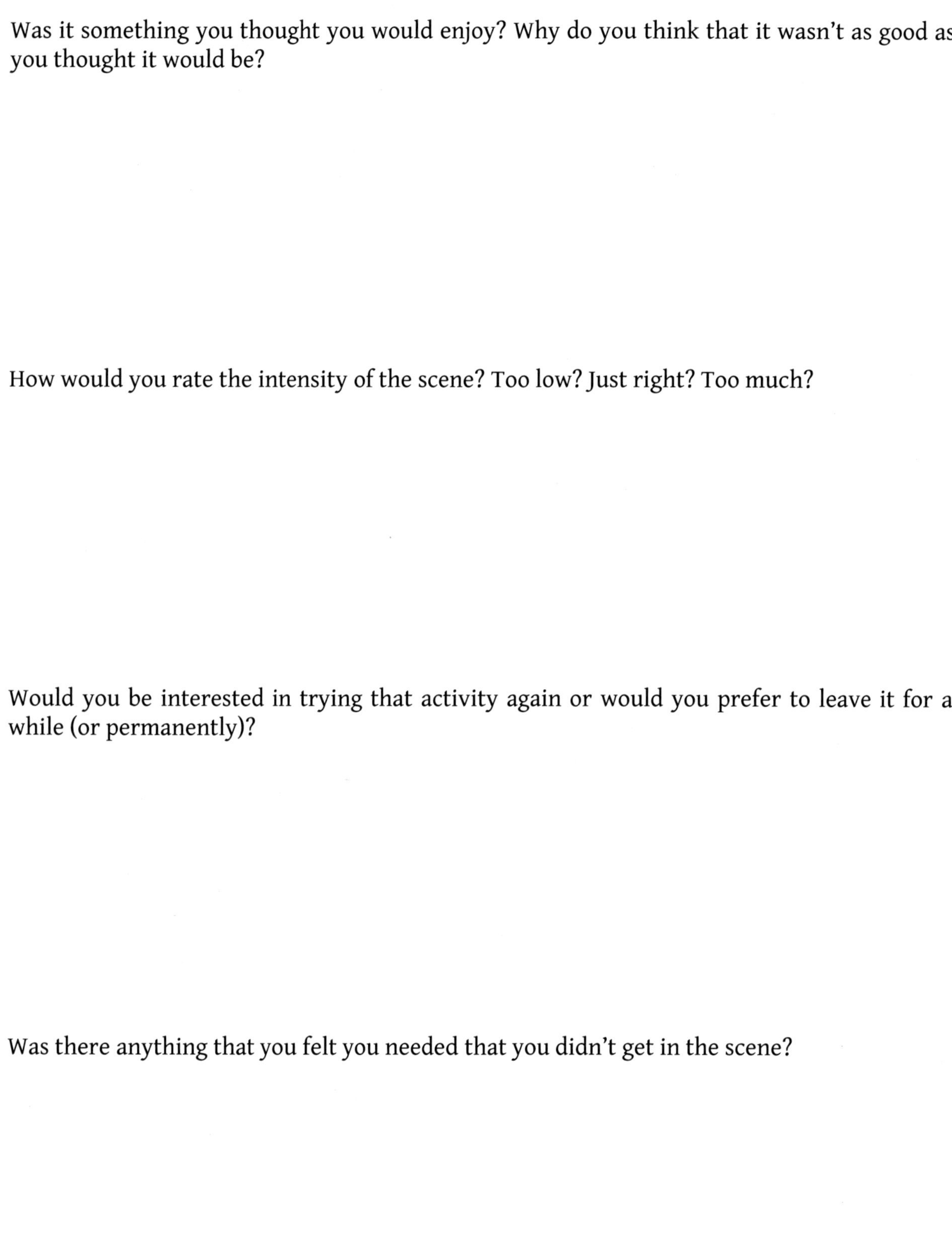

Was it something you thought you would enjoy? Why do you think that it wasn't as good as you thought it would be?

How would you rate the intensity of the scene? Too low? Just right? Too much?

Would you be interested in trying that activity again or would you prefer to leave it for a while (or permanently)?

Was there anything that you felt you needed that you didn't get in the scene?

How do you think the scene went overall?

Did you find that the aftercare was sufficient? Did you drop?

Name one thing you would change for next time and one thing you would like to keep the same.

Feel free to add any questions that you think are important. Remember that BDSM isn't just a physical experience, it's a mental and emotional one too. Make sure you address all of these aspects when you have your scene review. Even though it may be hard, it is really important, to be honest with your partner, otherwise, they may end up doing things you don't enjoy inadvertently.

18 EXPLORING BONDAGE:

BONDAGE SAFETY

Bondage is the art of restraining a person, limiting their movement, and making them feel helpless. It's that feeling of helplessness, of having no control, leaving the "real" world behind and being completely at the mercy of the one tying that so many people find appealing about it.

Over my years of personal and professional BDSM, I've tied and bound more people than I can count. Bondage is probably the #1 element of BDSM that is requested for scenes. I have to really think hard to recall BDSM scenes or sessions that haven't included at least some sort of bondage. Rope, cuffs, plastic wrap, hoods, blindfolds, gags - all of these contribute to the feelings of helplessness that so many bottoms crave.

I've been told that the appeal is that they can let go, explore their fantasies because they are no longer in charge. They aren't doing these things, I'm doing it to them. Of course, everything is heavily negotiated first and I don't do things that haven't been approved by my partner first (either because they have asked for the activity, agreed to it, or we are in a consensual non-consent style relationship).

Bondage safety, then, includes both physical safety as well as mental safety. Bondage can be a very intense experience for people. That loss of control over their bodies can bring out some strong emotions. I've known more than one person who has found bondage to be a cathartic experience.

If you haven't already read the chapter Impact and Pain Play Safety, or you're not clear on some of it, please go back and read it. There is a good deal of important information that will also apply to bondage safety. This chapter is intended to build on that one, adding specific information that you need to know before getting into bondage.

Physical Safety in Bondage

There are a number of ways that we can make bondage as safe as possible. In BDSM, we need to understand that nothing is ever 100% safe, but we can reduce risks and take appropriate safety precautions. Done properly, most bondage will be a relatively safe activity (not including edge play activities like rope suspension).

The first rule of bondage safety is to *never* leave a bound person alone. Ever. Not even for a second. Not to answer the door. Not to answer the phone in the other room. Not because it seems hot. NEVER.

There has been more than one news story about a person being left alone in bondage, having a medical emergency and the top returning too late to assist them. Too many people have died while left alone in bondage, let's not add to that number.

An important aspect of safety is to be careful that we aren't interfering with breathing or placing pressure on the throat. Suffice to say that anything which goes around or across the throat should be designed for it, that breathing and blood flow should not be restricted.

Do not ever tie off something that is attached to the throat. So don't attach a rope to a collar, then tie that rope to the bed. It can put pressure on the throat without you being aware of it. Never tie a collar, neck rope, etc to the ceiling with the bottom standing (I've seen it done), that's just asking for trouble.

Of course, the worst possible combination is restricted breathing, bondage and a bottom who is left alone. I personally knew someone who suffered the tragic consequences of this combination. Note I said knew. He was engaged in solo bondage play that involved a hood. I don't know all the details of what happened, but I do remember that the funeral shocked and devastated my local kink community.

Falling is another serious issue. Over the years of acting as a Dungeon Monitor (DM) for various parties, I've seen more injuries directly related to falling in bondage than all other injuries combined. Additionally, falling in bondage was responsible for the most serious injuries I've seen as well.

Never have someone whose arms are bound standing up without also having them secured to something to break a potential fall. I have seen a bottom lose multiple teeth, break her nose and jaw, as well as a number of other, less significant injuries because she fainted while bound and the top hadn't secured her so she couldn't fall. The top in question made a simple mistake that anyone could have. This wasn't a case of negligence or extreme play, it was a typical rope scene gone wrong.

Tying the feet and legs together, while a bottom is standing is a bad idea as well. This can cause them to easily lose their balance and fall. If they have their arms free, they may be able to break their fall, but it's still a fall.

It is a top's responsibility to look after the bottom. We have rendered them helpless, so take on the responsibility of caring for them. It is very important that you have a realistic understanding of your skill level and not play above it.

While it may seem like a good idea to have a bottom tied up and walking around in high heels, the risks are not worth it. Trust me, I learned this one from having a bound bottom stand for just a moment. It was a moment too long and one I regret to this day. Thankfully, a lump on the head and some soreness were the only injuries, but it shouldn't have happened.

Nerve damage is another serious consideration when engaging in rope bondage. It is a somewhat common injury in shibari style bondage, where ropes are wrapped around the body and often suspension is involved.

People who are new to bondage see things in images and try to recreate it without understanding the technical stuff. Or they see porn images, which may have been done by someone as new as they are.

There are a few precautions you need to take to avoid nerve damage in rope. Do not tie over the inside part of joints. I know this is a hard one to avoid since we want to tie wrists together, right? The key here is placing the wrists so that the soft undersides are together. Have the bottom offer the wrists with their palms together, almost in a prayer style position. This protects the part of the wrists where the nerves are closest to the surface.

You will notice that most cuffs, whether leather, vegan, metal or other materials are generally fairly wide. This width helps protect the wrists or ankles from nerve damage. It's also the reason that handcuffs are dangerous and generally not a good idea. Anything that is rigid and cuts into the wrist should not be used for bondage, especially with a bottom who struggles.

If you decide to pursue shibari or other more elaborate bondage, you will learn about other nerves that are exposed or close to the surface that you need to look out for.

In general terms, you want to look out for weakness in the hands (or affected limb) and pain, especially pain that radiates from one spot (so, if pain starts in the wrist and shoots down into the fingers). If your bottom experiences either of these things, it's best to undo the bondage and wait for things to get back to normal.

Fainting, which we talked about a bit with falling, is another hazard. There can be any number of reasons that people fall, including not eating or drinking enough, having alcohol or recreational drugs involved, and locking the knees while standing.

Finally, you should have a plan for emergency situations. What happens if there is a fire? An earthquake? If the bottom has a seizure? Anything can happen during a scene, so you should be prepared. Having paramedic shears on hand is a good idea (they have the nib at the end to prevent cutting skin). I also have a gadget that is intended to cut seat belts, I find that these make it easier to cut rope because it is sometimes too thick for scissors. Cuffs and shackles can be undone quickly, just make sure you have the key handy (around your neck is ideal) if you're using the locking type.

A Note on Knives

Knives are not an ideal tool for cutting rope. The long blade and pointed end can easily injure the bottom or the top. They can slip and cut both people, not just rope. This is not what you want to be using in an emergency situation.

Knives may "look cool" but they are not a good idea. If you are doing a planned scene where you cut things with a knife, that's one thing. Relying on one in the event you need to cut rope or restraints is just asking for trouble.

Do yourself and your bottom a favour, invest in a proper pair of shears (not regular scissors) or a seat belt cutter. You may lose cool points, but you will gain in real safety.

Normal Post-Bondage Stuff

There are a number of things that can happen after a good bondage scene that can be worrisome to a novice that aren't really a big deal. You probably don't have to worry about these things at all, but they may make for an awkward social situation from time to time.

Rope marks are probably the most likely after effect and generally aren't something you need to worry about. Rope marks that last longer than a few hours may indicate that the bondage was too tight, but it may not. Rope marks are seen in suspension bondage, especially for newer bottoms. The weight loaded onto the rope can cause small blood vessels to break, essentially a bruise (but they generally show up as red).

More typical bruises can happen if a knot digs into the skin. It could be the result of other play that was combined with the bondage. It could even happen with uncomfortable positioning where a bunch of rope digs into soft skin. Bruises can also happen with cuffs, especially metal shackles. Metal is a lot more unforgiving than rope or leather.

Both of those things, rope marks and bruises, are much more likely if the bottom struggles against the restraints. If you have a bottom who likes to struggle, it may be wise to use softer things like leather cuffs or straps for bondage. Alternately, you can simply do bondage in such a way that they are not able to move or struggle much.

It is also totally normal for the bottom to wake up the next day and have sore muscles. Doubly so if they were struggling against the bondage. Like a workout, bondage usually feels great while it's happening, you have endorphins flowing and don't realize how hard you are pushing your body. The next day, you pay the price for the fun.

Emotional Safety

Bondage, like many kinks, can be mild or extreme. There is something about bondage, though, that seems to affect us deeply in ways that other kinks don't. It takes away freedom, renders you helpless. Those are often viewed as positives when done within the context of a consensual kink relationship. It also leaves a person very vulnerable.

The top can do what they want, the bottom is in no position to stop them. Many of the professional submissives I know refuse to engage in bondage until they've had a few sessions with the person, so they can feel them out. Lifestyle submissives and bottoms often follow the same rule, limiting play with new partners to ones they can walk away from.

Another option, if you are trying bondage with a new partner or are engaging in more casual play, is to only do bondage at play parties, until you get to know and trust your partner more. Play parties should have a DM on hand who can step in during a worst-case scenario.

Playing while stressed or otherwise upset can bring out a lot of emotional trauma. You may not even realize how upset you were until tied up. It's one thing to play with the idea of cathartic release in mind, another to have it creep up on you unexpected. It's not unheard of for people to just start crying or freaking out during bondage scenes. If it happens, remove the bondage, give comfort, and offer to talk. The bottom may not know why they are crying, so don't pressure and don't assume it's you.

Ideally, we would only play when things are perfect. Enough sleep, food, no stress, no worries about money, the kids, etc. Sadly, that perfect world doesn't exist for most people. We have stressful jobs or bad days or the dog won't behave... The best we can do is be aware that these things may come up during a scene (bondage or no). We can try to push them to the back of our minds, but that may not always work. If that happens and the scene just isn't working, say so. Both tops and bottoms can have life interfere with play, we are all human and it happens. Your partner will be happier that you said something, rather than breaking down part way through a scene.

You should avoid doing new or strenuous bondage if you haven't slept properly, eaten properly, or are too stressed out. Save those scenes for another day when you're up to it. You don't have to not do BDSM, just tone it down and do something you're more comfortable with.

I know that's a lot to take in. Bondage, like the rest of BDSM, is a full-contact sport. There are risks. There are also rewards. I've written these chapters on safety because I want you to have many more rewards than risks.

19 EXPLORING BONDAGE: CHECKLIST

Bondage is a great activity in that it can stand alone - a scene can be a bondage scene and doesn't need to include any other elements - or it can be a part of a scene that has many different activities involved. For your first exploration into bondage, the focus should be the bondage itself. Enjoy some sensual or sexual play (if that's on the table) along with it, but really feel the restraint and how it adds to a scene. Notice how it shifts the power, even if you aren't specifically playing with power exchange.

Some bondage activities are simple and can be done with little to no instruction or investment, these are indicated by a ✪. Others require a specific purchase or some skill to accomplish and are marked with a 🕮. Finally, some bondage techniques are potentially dangerous and should be learned through in person instruction and practice. These are indicated by a ⚐.

How to Use the Checklist

You may find it easiest to photocopy this list or download it from my website at www.MsMorganThorne.com if you prefer to do it online or print it out yourself. Of course, you're more than welcome to fill out this one right here in the book if you want to keep things all in one place.

Both or all partners should fill out this checklist, to gauge interest in activities and so that they are aware of what the other(s) are interested in. If you have multiple partners, each pairing should fill out a checklist, as what you are willing to explore with one partner may be different than what you are willing to explore with another.

Make sure you indicate your experience, if any, with each activity. Again, this is the beginning of a conversation, not the whole thing. Don't be afraid to ask a person how they learned, whether they were a top or bottom for that activity, etc.

If an activity does not apply to you for whatever reason, simply ignore it or write in **N/A**.

Use a **T** or **B** to indicate that you would be interested in topping or bottoming for an activity. If you're interested in doing both, simply write both letters in.

Rating scale for the checklist. Remember, if you haven't tried an activity, indicate your interest level in that activity. If you plan on having others involved directly in your play, indicate with an * which activities you would want to keep between you and your primary partner or the person you are filling this checklist out with.

- **NO** is a hard limit, something you are not interested in doing under any circumstances.
- **0** (zero) is a soft limit, something you aren't interested in doing, but may consider under specific circumstances and with specific negotiation.
- **1** (one) is something you aren't really interested in doing but will oblige if it's requested occasionally.
- **2** (two) is something that you're okay with doing but you don't really enjoy. You will do it if asked, to please your partner, or as a special reward.
- **3** (three) is something that you neither like nor dislike. You're up for it if your partner wants to, but it's not something you would miss if it didn't happen.
- **4** (four) is something you enjoy doing and wouldn't mind doing often.
- **5** (five) is something you really want to do, something you would like to do as often as possible.
- **?** is something you don't understand or are truly unsure about.

Explanations can be found online - but be careful what you search for, you may not like what you see!

Always remember that these checklists are not written in stone. You can change your checklist whenever you like. If you try something and it's not nearly as much fun as you thought it would be, change it's rating. If you didn't think you would like something but have warmed up to the idea, change it's rating. Don't forge to let your partner know about the change. These checklists are a great way to keep track of things and for spurring conversations, but most of us don't check them before each time we play. I recommend using pencil to fill out your checklist so that you can change it whenever you need.

There are blank spots at the end of each checklist. If there is something that fits this category that I haven't included, write it in! I've also done my best to keep the lists somewhat short, which means I've left out some of the more extreme activities. If you are interested in more extreme play, make sure you get educated on how to do it safely, including attending workshops and reading all you can on the subject.

Name: Date:

Bondage Activity	Experience Y/N	Rating NO, 1-5, ?	Top or Bottom
Arm Binders 🕮			
Bed Restraints 🕮			
Blindfolds ✪			
Breast Bondage 🕮			
Body Bags 🕮			
Bondage (Light) ✪			
Bondage (Heavy) 🕮 ⚐			
Bondage (Long Term) ⚐			
Bondage Bed 🕮			
Cages 🕮			
Cells or Closets ✪			
Chains ✪			
Chest Bondage 🕮			
Cock Bondage (Rope) 🕮			

Bondage Activity	Experience Y/N	Rating NO, 1-5, ?	Top or Bottom
Cock Bondage (Devices) 🕮			
Cock Bondage (Metal) 🕮			
Cock Bondage (Leather) 🕮			
Cock Bondage (Latex/Rubber) 🕮			
Cock Rings ✪			
Collars ✪			
Collars (Posture) 🕮			
Corsets 🕮			
Cuffs (Leather) ✪			
Cuffs (Metal) 🕮			
Escaping Bondage ✪ 🕮 ⚐			
Gags (Cloth) ✪			
Gags (Bit) 🕮			
Gags (Ball) 🕮			
Gags (Inflatable) 🕮			
Gags (Phallic) 🕮			

Bondage Activity	Experience Y/N	Rating NO, 1-5, ?	Top or Bottom
Gags (Tape) ✪			
Gags (Ring) 📖			
Gags (Medical) 📖 🏳			
Gags (Open Mouth) 📖			
Gas Masks 📖			
Hair Bondage 📖			
Handcuffs 📖			
Harness (Leather) 📖			
Harness (Latex/Rubber) 📖			
Harness (Rope) 📖			
Harness (Other) 📖			
Hidden Bondage (Under Clothing) 📖			
Hoods 📖			
Immobilization 📖 🏳			
Japanese Bondage (Kinbaku or Shibari) 📖 🏳			
Japanese Bondage (Hojojutsu) 📖 🏳			
Leg Binders 📖			

Bondage Activity	Experience Y/N	Rating NO, 1-5, ?	Top or Bottom
Manacles and Irons 🕮			
Mental Bondage ✪			
Mummification ✪			
Plastic Wrap ✪			
Restraints (Leather) ✪			
Restraints (Vegan) ✪			
Restraints (Other) ✪			
Scarves, Ties, Pantyhose, etc ✪			
Self Bondage 🕮			
Shoe Bondage 🕮			
Sleep Sacks 🕮			
Sleep Bondage 🕮			
Spreader Bars 🕮			
Stocks & Pillories 🕮			
Straight Jacket 🕮			
Straps 🕮			
Stress Positions 🕮 ⚐			

Bondage Activity	Experience Y/N	Rating NO, 1-5, ?	Top or Bottom
Suspension (Sex Swing) 🕮			
Suspension (Rope) 🕮 ⚐			
Suspension (Other) 🕮 ⚐			
Tape Bondage ✪			
Thumb cuffs 🕮			
Vacuum Bed 🕮 ⚐			
Zip Ties 🕮			

20 EXPLORING BONDAGE:

SCENE CREATION AND IDEAS

Bondage is one of those wonderful kinks that can be used as part of a scene, or as a scene all on its own. You will have to decide if you're going to try just bondage or bondage with a few other things.

Bondage Specific Safety Concerns

In addition to the previous chapter on Bondage Safety, there are specific things you should be aware of with different types of bondage. Many of these items will simply be that you need to get in-person instruction before attempting them, like rope suspension.

Rope suspension can be beautiful and artistic. However, the models and riggers that you see in photographs have practised and trained for years to do what they do. Yes, the bottoms need to be strong, flexible, and able to know what they can handle, since so much of what you see in photos is very hard on the body.

If that sort of bondage appeals to you, I encourage you to find a rope group in your community. These will be listed in the advanced training section too, but Rope Bite (open to all) and Hitchin' Bitches (woman/femme identified tops only) are both international organizations dedicated to rope education. Their websites would be a good place to start.

Breast bondage can be tricky. Binding the breasts puts a lot of pressure on them, which causes vascular constriction. It is wise to limit the amount of time that breasts are tightly bound because breast tissue contains a greater concentration of endocrine tissues. They carry lymphatic fluids, which are part of the immune system and play a major role in the removal of abnormal cells.

Tight breast bondage should be avoided if the bottom has breast implants. The added pressure of the bondage can cause the implant to burst or leak.

Bondage which wraps around the chest can also cause breathing problems. If you tighten rope when the person has exhaled, they may not be able to expand their chest during an inhale. This can lead to shallow breathing, which can lead to hyperventilating, panic, and not being able to catch one's breath. If you have the rope or other restraints around the chest, have the person take a deep breath before tightening the restraints. This way, there is enough room for the chest to expand with normal breathing.

Many people like the idea of long-term bondage or overnight bondage. Personally, I will not have a person bound if I am asleep or not able to pay attention to them. You may find that the risks are acceptable to you and your partner. If you decide to engage in either, make sure the bottom has an escape plan. A way to get out of the bondage in an emergency. Never include bondage that involves the throat if you can't pay 100% attention to the person the whole time (like when you're asleep).

Corsets are popular in the fetish community. I'm a big fan myself, being an avid tightlacer. Corsets should not interfere with breathing and should never cause pain. If a corset is doing either of those things, it should be loosened. If you would like to get into corseting, please make sure you are educated on how to measure yourself and how to buy a well-fitting, properly made corset.

Cock and ball bondage can range from a simple cock ring, to various devices, to elaborate rope. Tightness is going to determine the length of time that you can keep the cock and balls bound for. The tighter the bondage, the less time you should keep them bound. If there is ever shooting pain, they should be unbound. Do not twist the testicles, this can cause a medical emergency known as a torsion.

Mummification is typically done with plastic wrap. This is fun and easy to do, just wrap your partner! Keep in mind that plastic wrap is hot, especially when it's covering your entire body (or most of it). Keep times limited if you are in a hot climate or hot room. Make sure the bottom stays hydrated and watch for dangerous overheating.

It is also important that you ensure the bottom can breathe. Part of this is being able to inhale fully, as discussed above. The other is if you are using a hood or doing mummification, you need to ensure that the bottom has unobstructed access to air. Even if it's a straw in the mouth or nose, make sure that they can breathe.

When engaging in tape bondage, don't put things like duct tape directly on the skin. The adhesive can bond with skin, tearing it off when you remove the tape. It can also cause some intense allergic reactions, which could be serious if enough of the skin is covered. Use plastic wrap against the skin, then add the tape around it. You can also use "bondage tape" a product designed to stick to itself and do not have adhesive.

Zip ties present the same hazards as handcuffs, that of serious nerve damage. They may seem like a simple choice or an appropriate one for an interrogation scene, but be careful. A struggling bottom can cause a lot of harm without realizing it.

Finally, using household items, such as silk ties, scarves, pantyhose, etc. may seem like an easy bondage solution. However, many of these items can tighten up knots, especially if the bottom struggles against the bonds. When it comes time to untie them, you may not be able to. Don't use anything you wouldn't want to cut and be prepared with scissors or a seat belt cutter to do so.

Scene Creation

If you decide to incorporate other activities, stick to the 3-5 rule, including the bondage. If you try to cram too much into a scene, it won't work out very well. Focus on a few activities and make them really good. You may want to limit things to only 1 or two activities other than bondage, or stick to sensual/sexual play while one partner is bound.

Compatible activities rated 4/5 or higher:

Who will top? Who will bottom?

Compatible activities 3/5:

Who will top? Who will bottom?

What positions will the bottom be in?

Which activities are off the table (listed as 2/5 or lower)?

Will you combine other activities with bondage? If so, what activities?

Planning Your Scene

When planning a bondage scene, you have to think about what you have on hand, what your skills are, and what you're trying to achieve. It's a fairly simple matter to tie a person's hands to the headboard, much more difficult to bind them so they can't move.

Talk about positions. Figure out what will work for your scene and what the bottom can reasonably do. Strenuous positions won't be feasible for a long scene. There are some positions that some bottoms may never be able to do. You need to work with the capabilities of you and your partner to achieve a good scene.

If you are adding other activities to the bondage scene, keep them simple for the first few times. Maybe it's a bit of teasing, getting them really worked up until they beg for sex. Maybe it's a bit of light spanking or other pain play. Remember that the bondage is supposed to be the star of this show, you can always plan for more intense scenes later.

An important lesson to remember when planning the timing of your scene, it takes around half as long to untie a person as it took to tie them up. That works for most other forms of bondage as well. Cuffs are simple to unbuckle, but they still take a moment. Plastic wrap is easy, just cut it off, but you need to be careful not to cut the bottom too!

Jamie and Taylor's Bondage Negotiation

Returning to Jamie and Taylor, they've also decided to give bondage a try. They have agreed that they will try some simple bondage involving some silk scarves they picked up at the second-hand store.

As usual, Jamie will top and Taylor will bottom. They've agreed that Taylor will be tied spread eagle, face up on the bed, with the possibility of being turned over if Jamie wants to. They've also agreed that they will do a bit of sensation play, mostly caressing and light touch. Taylor really liked the nipple clamps and has requested those, as well as a blindfold.

Once again, they will end the scene with sexual activity, with Taylor still bound during this part of the scene. Their safe words and other aspects remain the same as their other scenes. They gather their gear and safety supplies and head to the bedroom.

The Bondage Scene

Getting used to this BDSM thing, neither Jamie nor Taylor are really nervous getting started. They both strip nude, thinking that this will be easier. They start kissing and fall to the bed. Jamie grasps one of Taylor's wrists and guides it to the corner of the bed. Grabbing a silk scarf, Jamie secures Taylor's wrist to the bed frame. This is repeated until all four of Taylor's limbs are secure.

Jamie begins by stroking and caressing Taylor's body, getting both of them excited. Jamie tweaks Taylor's nipples and reaches for the clamps. Once firmly attached, Jamie turns and grabs the blindfold, placing it on Taylor's eyes.

Taylor is now bound and can not see. Every touch is amplified. Even Jamie's breath feels like electricity across the skin. Both partners are very aroused. Jamie continues to tease Taylor for a while, eventually removing the nipple clamps and enjoying Taylor's yelps.

They move on to sexual play, where Taylor strains against the bonds while writhing in pleasure. When they are done, Jamie unites Taylor's hands without incident, but the knots on Taylor's ankles just won't give. Taylor starts to feel claustrophobic and becomes a bit upset. Jamie tries to stay calm, reassuring Taylor and looking on the bedside table for the shears. Luckily, Jamie is able to gently cut away the scarves before Taylor gets too freaked out.

They cuddle in bed, Jamie trying to calm and reassure Taylor.

What Can We Learn?

This scene is the first where Jamie and Taylor have run into a problem. You never know how you will react in a situation until you're in it. Taylor didn't know that something like that would set off a feeling of panic. Jamie, as the top, did the right thing in staying calm and working quickly to fix the situation.

What do you think would have happened if Jamie had told Taylor to calm down and tried to undo the knots?

It could have turned out okay. It could have calmed Taylor but left Jamie frustrated when the knots wouldn't give. It could have sent Taylor over the edge into a full-on panic attack. It's impossible to say how people will react.

When you engage in bondage, you need to be willing to cut your bottom out of their bindings, if the need arises. Thankfully, that isn't really often. It is one of the hazards of playing with things not designed for bondage. I've had to cut more scarves and pairs of pantyhose used for bondage than rope. Actually, I don't think I've ever cut rope.

Panic While Bound

Panic can be a reaction to being bound. Many people will engage in bondage and be perfectly fine, but sometimes, things align in such a way that the bottom panics. This can be a difficult situation to handle safely.

If anything is restricting the bottom's breathing, it is the first thing you should fix. A panicking bottom with restricted breathing is a dangerous mix. Let them know you are aware of the problem and are moving to fix it. Tell them you're grabbing the scissors, untying the rope, etc.

If the bottom is wearing a blindfold or anything which restricts their vision, this should be the next priority for removal. Many people will panic when they can't see because they don't know what's coming next. Speak to them in a calm voice and tell them what you are doing. Say "I'm going to remove your blindfold, then I will remove the rest of the bondage". They need to hear it.

Gags should be the next item of priority. Even if they aren't interfering with breathing, it can feel like they are. They're also generally uncomfortable. Removing a gag can help restore calm.

Next, you need to remove the bondage in a manner which is safe to do. I don't suggest using scissors or anything sharp in this case because if the bottom thrashes or flails at the wrong time, you could both become injured. Untie or undo the bondage while speaking in a calm voice to the bottom, again telling them exactly what you are doing.

If you know how long it will take, tell them. "This is going to take about 5 minutes, I know you can make it" may help calm them a bit. They may yell at you to go faster. Don't give into the urge to untie really quickly. You will fumble with the knots or buckles, taking longer overall. Proceed calmly and with confidence (even if you don't feel calm or confident, you need to present that way to your bottom). You're not going to be helpful if you're panicking too.

21 EXPLORING BONDAGE: AFTERCARE AND SCENE REVIEW

Some people consider the scene over when the top starts removing the bondage. Others incorporate the removal of the bondage into the scene. Whichever route you choose to take, it's time to start shifting into aftercare mode (if you are planning on doing aftercare). At the very least, you will need to ensure that the bottom is in good condition and not injured.

Bondage Specific Aftercare

Aftercare for bondage can be exactly the same as it is with other activities. You may want to focus on massage with essential oils, massage oils or other lotions to help rejuvenate the skin and ease muscle tension.

During bondage, especially if it's strenuous or the bottoms struggles, they may have sore muscles the next day. Giving a good massage (look up techniques online, don't just do a half-assed rubdown), can help prevent some of the pain or stiffness that is considered to be normal after bondage.

If you're using natural fibre ropes like hemp or jute, you may want to use some moisturizer or oil on the skin. These types of ropes can draw moisture out of the skin, so replacing the lost moisture can be helpful. Besides, who doesn't want nice, soft skin?

You should always be aware of rope burn or marks. If the bottom has a lot of rope burn, it could be one of two things or a combination of the two. Synthetic rope can cause rope burn. If you're using nylon rope (please don't be using poly rope, it's not meant for bondage at all), this could be the problem. If you're using natural rope, it could be the type of rope - natural isn't always better. Sisal rope will leave splinters in the skin and is generally only used for very specific torture ties. Hemp or jute, which are ideal for bondage, can leave rope burn if you're pulling it too quickly across the skin. You do need to pull it pretty quickly to get rope burn, but it's possible. Sometimes it's a combination of the material of the rope and how quickly you're pulling it.

Place your hand between the bottom and the rope when you're pulling it through a knot or friction. This will protect the bottom and you will get instant feedback about what's causing the burn.

If rope burn does occur, treat it as you would any other injury. If the skin is broken, use appropriate first aid. If it's just irritated, you can rub some lotion on it or leave it, whatever the bottom prefers.

Bruising from tight restraints is hard to do anything for after the fact, but an ice pack may help keep it to a minimum. Some people find that arnica gel or products containing arnica may help with bruising.

Make sure the bottom has some water to drink. The top too, for that matter. Bondage can be hard work, and you both may be dehydrated.

Many bottoms will want a blanket after bondage. The bondage itself may have been keeping them warm, as in plastic wrap bondage. The exertion of holding a pose may have kept them warm or distracted but now they are cold. It is wise to have a blanket or sweater on hand for this.

Some people find coiling rope (or cleaning other restraints) to be a good way to come down from a bondage scene. Some leave it up to the bottom to do, others prefer to do it themselves. I've already expressed my preference to do these things myself, both because I'm very particular about how my rope is coiled (and how my other toys are cleaned) because I can examine it for flaws or damage, and it gives me time to focus and come back to reality.

Reviewing the Scene

Once again, you may want to do a scene review right after or wait a few days. Getting in the habit of talking about your scenes is a good idea - it doesn't always have to be this formal, but having a conversation about it can be helpful.

You may want to consider whether you added other activities or just stuck to bondage. Was this the right choice for you? Will you do the opposite next time? Did things go smoothly? Consider these things as you answer the following questions, which you should be getting used to by now.

What parts of the scene did you enjoy? What was your favourite? Why?

How did those parts of the scene make you feel? Why do you think that is?

Were those parts things you had highly rated? Were there any pleasant surprises (things you weren't sure about but really enjoyed)?

Was there a part of the scene that you didn't enjoy?

Was it something you thought you would enjoy? Why do you think that it wasn't as good as you thought it would be?

How would you rate the intensity of the scene? Too low? Just right? Too much?

Would you be interested in trying that activity again or would you prefer to leave it for a while (or permanently)?

Was there anything that you felt you needed that you didn't get in the scene?

How do you think the scene went overall?

Did you find that the aftercare was sufficient? Did you drop?

Name one thing you would change for next time and one thing you would like to keep the same.

Feel free to add any questions that you think are important. Remember that BDSM isn't just a physical experience, it's a mental and emotional one too. Make sure you address all of these aspects when you have your scene review. Even though it may be hard, it is really important, to be honest with your partner, otherwise, they may end up doing things you don't enjoy inadvertently.

22 EXPLORING SEXUALITY & SEXUAL TABOO: ETHICAL NON-MONOGAMY

Society teaches us that monogamy is the standard relationship model. Some people will claim it's the only correct model. Others say it's oppressive. As usual with these sorts of things, the answer will be different for everyone.

Some people are just wired to be monogamous. That's perfectly okay. There is nothing wrong with wanting sexual and emotional fidelity between you and your partner. We won't be talking too much about monogamy since it is the dominant relationship structure in most of the world today.

This section is not solely focused on non-monogamy, so if it's something you're not interested in or that you're already experienced in, feel free to skip to the checklist. It contains a number of activities that will guide you through exploring a number of different aspects of sexuality.

A Note on Cheating

Many kinksters engage in what is known as ethical non-monogamy. There are many different flavours of non-monogamy, but the thread that runs through all of them is that everyone involved must be consenting to the situation.

Consent is taken very seriously in BDSM communities. Without that, what we do is abuse. Without consent, we are monsters.

There is also an equally important theme of trust and communication. If we don't trust our partners, we can't do what we do. We can't trust them to heed safe words, to take our safety seriously, to not recant their consent after the fact (although consent can be removed at any time during play).

Cheating breaks all these rules. Someone who cheats is untrustworthy. They do not respect their partner's boundaries. They don't have the courage to talk to their partner about ethical non-monogamy. Or, if they have, their partner said no and they want to do it anyway.

None of these are good things. None of them are qualities that kinksters want in a partner.

I've never seen a community of people feel so passionately about not cheating as kinksters. They almost all condemn the behaviour. Few would willingly or knowingly play with a cheater. They don't think much of excuses either, from what I've seen.

Sexless marriage? Vanilla spouse? Different kinks? Talk it out. Decide if you can do ethical non-monogamy or whether you should end the relationship (because there's a good chance it will end when you get caught cheating).

Your definition of cheating may differ from mine, but I consider any activity that you don't want to tell your spouse about to be cheating. Talking to someone online? If you can't tell your partner, it's cheating. Kissing someone? If you can't tell your partner it's cheating.

Ethical non-monogamy can be hard. Talking to your partner about it can be hard. It's an important step to take if you want to be non-monogamous. It's important that everyone involved is consenting.

Sexual Monogamy, Poly Play

One twist that some monogamous kinky people put on their relationships is that they may engage in non-sexual play with others. The only time they do sexual play is with each other exclusively.

If this is a style of monogamy you are interested in exploring, it is important to have a discussion about what non-sexual play involves for you. What I see as nonsexual play may be sexual for you. What you find non-sexual, I may find deeply sexual.

Communication with your partner is paramount. Many people who engage in this style of monogamy choose to only play at parties where their partner is present. This eliminates any suspicion of lying or inappropriate play.

Of course, it can be a bit tricky if you have different schedules, don't feel comfortable playing in front of your partner or for any other reason. Once again, honesty and communication are essential.

Mono/Poly

Another configuration is mono/poly, where one partner is monogamous and the other is polyamorous or allowed to have other partners.

This arrangement can take many different forms. It could be part of a power exchange dynamic where the dominant is allowed multiple submissives but the submissives are only allowed the one dominant.

It could be a case of one partner being vanilla and unable or unwilling to indulge the other's kinks themselves. They come to an arrangement where the kinky partner is allowed to have certain types of play with other partners. This takes clear communication and an effort to learn about kink by the vanilla partner, whether they engage or not.

Sometimes, things happen in life that leaves one partner without a sex drive or incapable of sex. In this case, a possible solution is to allow the still sexual partner to engage with others, whether in other relationships or “friends with benefits” style. Once again, this is a bit of a delicate situation and one that should be handled carefully to preserve the dignity of both partners.

Polyamory

Polyamory or poly for short is where people engage in multiple relationships. These are generally full relationships, including dating, spending quality time together, as well as sex. There are a number of different styles of poly, but they all involve having multiple relationships, not just lots of sexual partners.

Hierarchical Poly

This is where you would have a “primary” partner, perhaps a spouse or long-term relationship partner, as well as other “secondary” relationships. It is understood that the primary relationship would come first and be protected over and above the secondary relationships.

Often, people who engage in this style of poly will have a primary relationship and have secondary relationships with others who also have primary partners. It’s a bit easier to come second when you already have someone with whom you come first.

Egalitarian Poly

The opposite of hierarchical poly. All relationships are considered equal, rather than one having more importance than another. Generally, it elevates the sexual autonomy of the individual and emphasizes sexual equality.

Relationship Anarchy

Relationship anarchy is a poly style where all relationships are considered to be on equal footing. There are no primary or secondary partners, just partners. There may not be a strict distinction between sexual and non-sexual relationships, only what the people involved agree too. It can be viewed as a more extreme version of egalitarian poly.

Often people who practice relationship anarchy and hierarchical poly do not agree with each other's approach to poly and don't date.

OPP

OPP stands for "One Penis Policy" or "One Pussy Policy" and basically states that the partner(s) may seek out same-sex partners, but not opposite-sex partners. This is often seen in relationships that involve a heterosexual man and a bisexual or pansexual woman. She is allowed to date women and may be expected to share those partners with her male partner.

There are other configurations of this too, where a dominant may have a harem of submissives, all of the same gender, who are expected to interact with the dominant as well as each other.

Poly-fidelity

Poly-fidelity refers to a group of partners who are sexually exclusive to each other. Often this is seen as a closed triad - three people in a relationship together who do not date anyone else. It can also refer to larger groups of people, who are sexually active with each other but not with people outside of the group.

Open Relationships

Open relationships are the same as poly relationships for some people, for others, there is a distinction. Open relationships generally mean that the people involved are free to seek out sexual encounters (or kink encounters) but not engage in full on relationships. Sex is fine, but a dinner date is crossing the line.

Where the line falls is going to be different for everyone, so should be discussed ahead of time.

DADT

Don' ask don't tell (DADT) is a bit of a grey area. Ideally, it's where partners are free to engage others for sex but their primary partner doesn't want to know about it. This can be seen in some mono/poly relationships.

Many people will not engage with someone with a DADT arrangement since it can be hard to figure out if they actually have permission or they're just cheating.

SWINGING/SWAPPING

Swinging has gained a lot of popularity in the past decade - or at least a lot of visibility. It is an activity that is usually engaged in as a couple, finding another couple to swap spouses/partners with. Sometimes the result is group sex, other times it's separate.

Swinging can include a range of activities from having sex in the same room as others to only female partners having sexual contact, to having sex with other couples in the same room or separate areas.

It should be noted that the social rules of swing culture tend to be a bit more permissive of touching than BDSM culture. Due to this difference, the two groups don't always get along. People primarily involved in swing also tend to view BDSM as foreplay, while people primarily involved in BDSM view it as it's own thing, with sex optional. These differences can clash when the two groups are together, although it is improving as more people get involved in both cultures.

SOFT SWAP

Soft soft swap covers a range of activities, so will take a bit of talking about. It usually is considered to involve activities that don't involve penetration or PIV sex (keeping in mind that most swing communities involve hetero couples). Many couples start with soft swap, some trying a full swap (sexual intercourse) at a later time.

CUCKOLDING & CUCKQUEANING

These are more specific sexual fantasies that include non-monogamy from one partner and include a hefty dose of humiliation as well. The cuckold or cuckquean is sexually humiliated by their partner who sleeps with others, either in front of them or tells them in exact detail after. Many cucks have a "cleaning up" fantasy, where they use their mouths to clean the sexual fluids of the other person from their partner.

HOT WIFING

I'm not sure if there is a name for a person who proudly shares their male partner, but the sharing of a female partner, without humiliation, is often called hot wifing. This can be done without any power exchange, simply because one partner enjoys watching the other have sex with other people. It can also be done by a dominant who lends their submissive to others for sexual use.

Other Non-Monogamous Relationship Styles

There are, of course, other styles of non-monogamous relationships but these are the main categories you will come across.

If you are interested in exploring non-monogamy, you first should narrow down what style of relationship you would like to try. Even if you try something else later or try it and find it's not for you, the style of relationship is going to influence how you negotiate the rules and permissions needed to make sure things go as smoothly as possible.

Jealousy and Compersion

We are all familiar with the concept of jealousy. It's a terrible feeling, the resentment of a perceived rival, feeling inferior, feeling ignored by your partner. It happens to everyone at some point.

When you're involved in non-monogamous relationships, jealousy happens from time to time and can be difficult to deal with. Honesty is very important here. If you are feeling jealous, understanding why is a very important step to overcoming it.

Are you feeling jealous because your partner is having more dating success than you are? Is it because they seem to be paying more attention to their new partner? Are they neglecting your rules or other boundaries?

There can be many reasons for feeling jealous, some more justified or understandable than others. Talking to your partner calmly, explaining why you are jealous and working together to find a solution is the best way to approach it. Whether that means you set aside extra time together to have a date night, your partner slows down on dating others for a bit, or they apologize for breaching agreements and make amends will be determined by the situation.

Maybe the rules and boundaries you both set up before trying non-monogamy are unrealistic. There are a lot of things which may seem reasonable to people who are inexperienced, but once you start dating others, you find it's not feasible. If that is the case, it's best to renegotiate as soon as you realize the rules are a problem, ignoring or breaking them will only cause resentment.

Dating others can seem exciting and exotic, especially if you've been together for a while and spend most of your time together doing mundane things. Dealing with the kids, household chores, finances, etc is pretty boring compared to the shiny new lover you see on weekends. If this is causing you problems in your existing relationship, you may need to set aside time specifically for reconnecting. Have someone watch the kids and spend a romantic evening together. Do something special, go on vacation - it doesn't really matter what you do, as long as you're doing it together.

New Relationship Energy (NRE)

NRE or new relationship energy is that wonderful time at the start of a relationship where you can't get enough of each other. They're perfect, not because they really are perfect but because you don't know them well enough to see their flaws. You're infatuated.

This can result in neglecting your already established relationships. If this happens, it's not unusual for jealousy to also happen. Imagine how you would feel if your partner was obsessing over someone else and neglecting you.

Learning to balance NRE and existing relationships can be difficult. It's a bit like walking a tightrope sometimes. Hopefully, your partner is understanding and won't mind a bit of infatuation, as long as you don't totally neglect them.

Compersion

Compersion is the opposite of jealousy. It is finding joy in another person's happiness. This is a feeling that many poly people have when their existing partner finds happiness with someone else (providing they are still acting appropriately towards the existing partner).

It can be an unusual feeling, but it's one we are probably all familiar with in some manner, we just didn't know what it was called. Think about watching a loved one open gifts on their birthday. You're happy when they get something they really wanted, you find joy in their joy. That's compersion.

It is possible to feel this in relation to your partner enjoying a relationship that doesn't involve you. You want to see your partner happy and they are.

Non-Monogamy as Fantasy Only

There are some people who are not comfortable with non-monogamy. Whether it's because of their childhood programming that says you can only have one romantic and sexual partner at a time or because they just aren't into it, it doesn't really matter.

They may, or their partner may find the idea but not the reality of non-monogamy hot. There are a few ways you can explore this theme without actually involving others.

Swing clubs are great for these fantasies. You can go and try a soft swap, negotiating the parameters you feel comfortable with. If that's too much, you can always just enjoy the exhibitionism of having sex in front of others or be voyeurs and watch others have sex.

Going to a swing club and not actively participating is usually okay, at least at the few that I've been to. As long as you are respectful of others, no one should complain.

You can also play around with flirting with other people. It's best to be upfront that flirting is all you're up for right now. Your partner might find it's a turn on to have such a desirable partner. Or they may find that it sets off the jealousy alarms in their head and any sort of non-monogamy will be in fantasy only.

We will talk about how to incorporate role play into this fantasy in the chapter Exploring Role Play.

You can also involve others, either real people or fantasy characters, by engaging in some dirty talk. Talk about what you would like to do to someone else, what you would like them to do to you. If you both have good imaginations, you can have quite the adventure!

Considerations for Negotiation

There are things that should be taken into account if you are planning on involving others in your play or relationships. Here is a list of things you may want to consider. There's a lot of them, so use what applies and disregard the rest.

- What style of non-monogamy will you engage in?
    - Will your outside relationships be sexual only? More involved?
    - Will you be engaging in sexual or non-sexual play?
        - How do you define non-sexual play?
- What activities are acceptable, which ones aren't?
- What safer sex practices will you observe?
    - How will you handle an STI? Or STI scare?
    - Is pregnancy a risk?
    - How will you mitigate that risk?
    - How will you handle it if it happens?
    - How will you handle it if safer sex precautions fail?
- What boundaries do you need for your own emotional health?
    - Are these different from safety boundaries?
    - What will you do if you discover an emotional boundary because it was breached (you didn't know it existed until you or your partner did something to cross it)?
- Will you both be allowed to engage with others?
    - Members of any gender or just one?
- What are the rules?
- Do you need to seek your partner's approval before a date?
- Can your partner veto someone?
    - What conditions can they veto?
- Do you need to tell your partner before a date?
    - Before sex?

- If you are dating within your social circle, is anyone off limits?
- What happens if you hate your partner's partner?
- Will these boundaries and rules apply to everyone you date? Only some relationships?
    - How will you decide the difference?
- How will you handle (primary) relationship health?
    - Will you have check-ins where you talk about how things are going?
- How will you adjust the rules as things change?
- How will you handle it if one partner asks for a rule or boundary that the other doesn't agree with or finds stifling?
- Will your partners meet?
    - Do you want them to be friends, if possible?
    - Do you want them to be lovers, if possible?
- What are your goals for non-monogamy? What do you want to get out of it?
- What will you do if you run into trouble in your primary relationship?
    - One partner has health issues?
    - One partner breaks trust?
    - One partner loses interest?
    - Other issues?
- How will you handle dating and childcare (if applicable)?
    - Take turns having dates/looking after the kids?
    - Find a good babysitter?
- How will you handle bringing partners home?
    - Will you only engage outside of your home?
- Are there any activities that are reserved just for your primary partner?
    - What are they?
- How much time will be dedicated to outside partners?
- Are there times when the regular rules don't apply?
    - Will they be more or less restrictive?
- Are you going to try taking things slowly or jump in with both feet?
    - What does that look like to you?
- What happens if one of you changes their mind?
- What happens if one of you doesn't follow the rules?
- What happens if one of you falls in love with an outside partner?
- What if you are on separate dates and end up at the same place/party?
- What happens if you can't agree on the fundamental rules of non-monogamy for you?

- How will you explain your relationship to others?
    - Will you tell your friends?
    - Family?
    - Kids?
    - Co-workers?

These are just some of the questions that you may want to consider before opening up your relationship. You may have other areas of concern that you need to include. Some of these may not apply to you.

No matter what, it is important to consider things from all angles before you open up your relationship, especially if you are new to non-monogamy. Spend as much time talking about it as you need to. Go only as fast as the slowest partner is comfortable with. Some people spend years thinking and talking about non-monogamy. For others, they know what they want and move more quickly.

Understand that it's not just you who gets to date others (unless you've agreed to a mono/poly relationship). Your partner is going to be dating others as well. Think about how that makes you feel and do your best to talk about and deal with any feelings of jealousy now, before you engage others.

It's not unusual for newly non-monogamous couples to have a lot of rules and restrictions that more experienced couples would never consider. That's okay, everyone starts somewhere. If you need a million rules to feel comfortable, that's fine. You probably will find that you're okay with many fewer once you have a bit of experience.

Write your rules and boundaries down but do it in a manner that is easy to change. Write it in pencil. Use a word processing document that you can easily change. Your rules won't stay the same once you get out into the real world of dating. You may need to add things you hadn't thought of, you may get rid of things you don't need.

Set aside some time to sit down and talk about the relationship and non-monogamy. Use this time to figure out if it's working for both of you or if things need to change. Relationships are dynamic, they don't just always stay the same. Be open to change and willing to make things work.

23 Exploring Sexuality & Sexual Taboo: Checklist

Sexuality is a fluid and interesting thing to explore. How you feel now may change drastically in the future or you may find that you are happy in your role and don't change that over time. Sexual taboo is different for everyone, although there are some fairly universal societal taboos that we can play with.

Not everyone is comfortable exploring in this area. Others will have this as a main focus for exploration, with everything else just window dressing. No matter which side you land on, it's always interesting to see what our taboos are and try to understand why they are so taboo.

Many of these activities involve non-monogamy. If you are strictly monogamous, simply skip those activities which do not apply or mark N/A in the field.

Please make sure you are familiar with safer sex practices, especially if you are engaging with multiple partners. If you need a refresher, take a look at the sexual safety section.

Most of these are activities anyone can do. These are marked with a ✪. Activities which take more negotiation and communication (likely because they involve other people) are indicated with a 🕮. High risk activities, both in terms of sexual health and potential emotional landmines are marked with ⚐.

How to Use this Checklist

You may find it easiest to photocopy this list or download it from my website at www.MsMorganThorne.com if you prefer to do it online or print it out yourself. Of course, you're more than welcome to fill out this one right here in the book if you want to keep things all in one place.

Both or all partners should fill out this checklist, to gauge interest in activities and so that they are aware of what the other(s) are interested in. If you have multiple partners, each pairing should fill out a checklist, as what you are willing to explore with one partner may be different than what you are willing to explore with another.

Make sure you indicate your experience, if any, with each activity. Again, this is the beginning of a conversation, not the whole thing. Don't be afraid to ask a person how they learned, whether they were a top or bottom for that activity, etc.

If an activity does not apply to you for whatever reason, simply ignore it or write in **N/A**. Use a **T** or **B** to indicate that you would be interested in topping or bottoming for an activity. If you're interested in doing both, simply write both letters in.

Rating scale for the checklist.

Remember, if you haven't tried an activity, indicate your interest level in that activity. If you plan on having others involved directly in your play, indicate with an * which activities you would want to keep between you and your primary partner or the person you are filling this checklist out with.

- **NO** is a hard limit, something you are not interested in doing under any circumstances.
- **0** (zero) is a soft limit, something you aren't interested in doing, but may consider under specific circumstances and with specific negotiation.
- 1 (one) is something you aren't really interested in doing but will oblige if it's requested occasionally.
- **2** (two) is something that you're okay with doing but you don't really enjoy. You will do it if asked, to please your partner, or as a special reward.
- **3** (three) is something that you neither like nor dislike. You're up for it if your partner wants to, but it's not something you would miss if it didn't happen.
- **4** (four) is something you enjoy doing and wouldn't mind doing often.
- **5** (five) is something you really want to do, something you would like to do as often as possible.
- **?** is something you don't understand or are truly unsure about.

Always remember that these checklists are not written in stone. You can change your checklist whenever you like. If you try something and it's not nearly as much fun as you thought it would be, change it's rating. If you didn't think you would like something but have warmed up to the idea, change it's rating. Don't forge to let your partner know about the change. These checklists are a great way to keep track of things and for spurring conversations, but most of us don't check them before each time we play. I recommend using pencil to fill out your checklist so that you can change it whenever you need.

There are blank spots at the end of each checklist. If there is something that fits this category that I haven't included, write it in! I've also done my best to keep the lists somewhat short, which means I've left out some of the more extreme activities. If you are interested in more extreme play, make sure you get educated on how to do it safely, including attending workshops and reading all you can on the subject.

Name: Date:

Sexuality & Sexual Taboo Activity	Experience Y/N	Rating NO, 1-5, ?	Top or Bottom
Anal Sex ✪			
Anal Plugs ✪			
Anal Plugs (in Public) ✪			
Chastity 🕮 ⚐			
Chastity Devices 🕮 ⚐			
Cock Rings ✪			
Cuckold 🕮 ⚐			
Cuckquean 🕮 ⚐			
Cybersex ✪			
Digital Penetration (Fingering) ✪			
Dirty Talk ✪			
Dildos ✪			
Double Penetration ✪ 🕮			
Edging ✪			
Ethical Non-Monogamy ✪ 🕮 ⚐			

Sexuality & Sexual Taboo Activity	Experience Y/N	Rating NO, 1-5, ?	Top or Bottom
Erotic Dance (Private) ✪ 🕮			
Erotic Dance (Audience) ✪ 🕮 ⚐			
Erotic Photos (Looking at) ✪			
Erotic Photos (Taking, Private) ✪ 🕮			
Erotic Photos (Taking, Posted Online) ✪ 🕮 ⚐			
Erotic Videos (Watching) ✪			
Erotic Videos (Making) ✪ 🕮			
Erotic Videos (Posted Online/Sold) ✪ 🕮 ⚐			
Exhibitionism (Friends) ✪ 🕮			
Exhibitionism (Strangers) ✪ 🕮			
Face Sitting ✪			
Fisting (Anal) 🕮			
Fisting (Vaginal) 🕮			
Forced Bisexuality 🕮			
Forced Masturbation ✪			
Forced Nudity (Private) ✪			
Forced Nudity (Public Sex Club/Dungeon) ✪ 🕮			

Sexuality & Sexual Taboo Activity	Experience Y/N	Rating NO, 1-5, ?	Top or Bottom
Forced Orgasms ✪			
Genital Sex ✪			
Genital Piercings (Have/Getting) 🕮 ⚐			
Given Away for Sex 🕮 ⚐			
Glory Hole 🕮 ⚐			
Group Sex 🕮 ⚐			
Hand jobs ✪			
Harems (With Other Subs/Bottoms) 🕮 ⚐			
Hook (Anal) ✪ 🕮			
Hook (Vaginal) ✪ 🕮			
Hot Wife 🕮 ⚐			
Kissing ✪			
Masturbation (Performative) ✪			
Masturbation (Mutual) ✪			
Nipple Play ✪			
Nipple Piercings (Have/Getting) 🕮 ⚐			
Nipple Clamps ✪ 🕮			

Sexuality & Sexual Taboo Activity	Experience Y/N	Rating NO, 1-5, ?	Top or Bottom
Nipple Weights ✪ 🕮			
Nipple Suction ✪ 🕮			
Opposite Sex Encounters			
Oral Sex ✪			
Orgasm Denial ✪			
Orgasm Control ✪			
Orgasm On Demand 🕮			
Orgies 🕮 ⚐			
Outdoor Sex ✪			
Pegging ✪			
Phone Sex ✪			
Polyamory ✪ 🕮 ⚐			
Post Orgasm Torture 🕮			
Public Exposure (Sex Clubs/Dungeons) 🕮			
Public Sex ✪ 🕮			
Queening ✪			
Ravishment Play (Rape Play) 🕮 ⚐			

Sexuality & Sexual Taboo Activity	Experience Y/N	Rating NO, 1-5, ?	Top or Bottom
Ravishment Play (Group) ⚐			
Rimming/Analingus ✪ 🕮			
Ruined Orgasms ✪ 🕮			
Same Sex Encounters			
Sex for Pay Fantasy 🕮			
Sex Doll 🕮			
Sex Slave 🕮			
Sex Toys ✪			
Sexual Deprivation (Temporary) ✪			
Sexual Deprivation (Long Term) 🕮			
Shared Sexually (With Friends) 🕮 ⚐			
Shared Sexually (With Strangers) ⚐			
Skinny Dipping ✪			
Slutty Clothing (Private) ✪			
Slutty Clothing (Public) 🕮			
Speculum (Anal) 🕮			
Speculum (Vaginal) 🕮			

Sexuality & Sexual Taboo Activity	Experience Y/N	Rating NO, 1-5, ?	Top or Bottom
Strap On (Wear) ✪			
Strap On (Suck) ✪			
Strap On (Penetrate) ✪			
Swallow Semen/Sexual Fluids ✪ 🕮			
Swap Partners 🕮 ⚐			
Swinging 🕮 ⚐			
Tantric Sex 🕮			
Teasing ✪			
Tease and Denial ✪			
Threesomes 🕮 ⚐			
Triple Penetration ✪ 🕮			
Unusual Insertions (Food, Objects, etc) ✪			
Vibrators ✪			
Voyeurism ✪			
Worship (Breast) ✪			
Worship (Cock) ✪			
Worship (Pussy) ✪			

Sexuality & Sexual Taboo Activity	Experience Y/N	Rating NO, 1-5, ?	Top or Bottom
Worship (Ass) ✪			

24 Exploring Sexuality & Sexual Taboo: Scene Creation and Ideas

A big part of the appeal of BDSM is the acceptance and exploration of sexual taboos. Many people have fantasies that they are afraid to tell anyone about, due to sex-negative conditioning during childhood that carries over into adulthood. They see depictions of BDSM and they see people unashamed of their sexual desires, even when 'out of the ordinary'.

Now, I don't want to paint the BDSM community as some bastion of sex-positivity and total acceptance. There are many unspoken rules that one needs to navigate. Sometimes, people can be pretty horrible to each other. Concepts of slut-shaming, misogyny, and other sex-negative attitudes are present in kink culture too - less prevalent than in the vanilla world, but still here. The members of the kink community are people, just like any other. Some will have rigid views on right and wrong that may not always align with yours.

We will look at the concept of multiple partners in its own chapter, chapter name. For now, I want to take a moment to talk about gender in the BDSM world.

Gender & BDSM

Gender is a social construct, distinct from sex. You may not agree, but it is the current belief of the majority of social scientists, psychologists, and most importantly in this instance, kinksters. You will come across many people who do not fit into the traditional gender moulds.

I won't go into a large amount of detail on this subject, but I will try to provide at least a basic understanding of what you may find, in the community or maybe even within yourself.

Gender, as many people understand it, consists of a binary. You are male or female. You are a man or a woman. This leaves out a growing number of people who don't identify strongly with these labels or find themselves with an identity different than the one they were assigned at birth. There are even some people who do not identify with any gender. We now refer to gender as a spectrum, to allow for all the wonderful variations that are possible.

These people are said to be part of the transgender spectrum. I would hope by this point, this book is published in late 2017, that we all understand what a transgender person is. They identify as a gender that is not the one they were assigned at birth, based on anatomy. The glossary has a number of definitions regarding the different identities - keep in mind that these are just general guidelines. Gender identity is an evolving concept, it is being refined and better understood as time goes on. I imagine that at least some of what I write here will be outdated in a few years.

There are other identities on the gender spectrum as well. As mentioned earlier, there are people who don't identify with any gender, we call them agender (the prefix "a" means "no" or "without"). Agender people may present as androgynous, a combination of genders may try out different gender identities or may simply continue expressing themselves as the gender they were assigned at birth. Whatever their choices in expression, this does not invalidate their gender identity.

Other people find that they alternate between feeling like a man and a woman (or other genders). They may choose to express themselves as one gender one day and the other the next day. They may continue to express themselves as the gender they were assigned at birth most of the time, only expressing the other parts of their identity when it is safe to do so. They may feel more comfortable with one gender and express themselves in that way most of the time.

A big thing here is safety. The BDSM community prides itself on being a safe space for gender exploration and acceptance. This is not always true - although many of us wish it was. Trans people may still feel unsafe in kink spaces. Let's try not to add to that, and work towards BDSM spaces being safe for everyone.

An important note here is that people on the trans spectrum are not, and should not be confused with cross-dressing. Cross-dressing is a fetish, a kink. It has little to do with gender identity - other than the person cross-dressing gets some sort of thrill out of wearing clothing usually associated with a gender they are not.

Sexual Taboo Specific Safety Concerns

The obvious one here is the risk of sexually transmitted infections (STIs). There are a number of safer sex precautions that you may wish to engage in to minimize risks. We will go over these briefly here and I encourage you to do some research if you are unfamiliar with anything mentioned here.

Overview of Safer Sex Practices

Condoms are the safe sex tool that people are most familiar with. If you plan on using condoms, understand their uses, limitations, and how to use one effectively. Condom sizing can be an issue for some people, so understand the signs of a condom that is too big (slips off or out of place during use) or one that is too small (cuts into the skin, causes discomfort). Condom companies offer a variety of sizes, so make sure you have one that is right for you.

Condoms can be used on toys, not just people. I prefer to cover my sex toys with condoms to make cleanup easier. This is also important if you are engaging in play with multiple people or doing anal play. Condoms are pretty stretchy, and if you don't need to worry about the comfort of a person, can be made to fit over any number of objects. I often place one over the head of my Hitachi Magic Wand, because it's been used on a number of different people. Obviously, toys need to be appropriately cleaned after each use, even if covered in a condom, but it helps cut down on the fluids that come in contact with the toy.

Condoms which are used to cover a toy can sometimes be referred to as "male" condoms. I prefer external condom, recognizing that they are used on people and objects that are not always male.

In contrast "female" condoms - again, internal condoms is a more appropriate term - are designed to sit inside the body with part of the condom remaining outside. There is a ring in each end, which is used during vaginal insertion so that it will sit against the cervix. If using this style of condom anally, the internal ring should be removed for comfort. A bonus of these condoms is that some of the condoms remain outside of the body, limiting genital to genital or genital to anal contact.

Dental dams are a sheet of latex or nitrile which can be placed against the genitals during oral sex or external contact with sex toys. If you can't find dental dams, you can cut open a latex or nitrile glove for a similar result.

Gloves are often used when digital (fingers/hands) genital contact will occur. For many people, they are a must for digital-anal contact. Once again, they help keep any mess under control and you don't have to worry as much about spreading bacteria.

Of course, condoms and gloves should be switched between partners, otherwise, STIs can be transmitted. Internal condoms are also good for MFF threesomes so that there is less swapping of condoms. Really, any configuration of people where there are multiple receptive partners and only one top.

You may hear the term "fluid bonded". This is when partners choose to forgo condoms with each other, usually after exchanging STI test results and establishing a committed relationship. If they have sexual contact with others, they will usually require that all normal safer sex practices be followed.

STI testing is also common in kink communities. How often it's done really depends on whether the person has multiple partners, whether their partner(s) have multiple partners, etc. Most people in open or poly arrangements get tested every 3-6 months.

It is important to remember that your STI test results give you a snapshot in time. You may not have any STIs when the test was done, but if you have had sexual contact with anyone after that, those results may not still hold true.

What STI tests do is allow us to know our status. If we have an STI, we can seek treatment. We can inform partners so that they can give real, informed consent to sexual activity. We can take precautions to prevent further spread of the STI.

Other Safety Concerns

Anal sex is a very popular activity but it is often done in a way that results in pain, tears, bleeding and other issues. Going slow with anal is important, allowing the body to relax and accept larger objects (toys, fingers, penises, etc). The other is to use lots of lube. If you think you have enough lube, you don't - add more. Using a good quality lube will mean it stays slippery longer so you won't have to refresh it as often.

Lube itself can be an issue. Do not use oil based lubes (coconut oil, etc) if you are using latex barriers. Oil breaks down latex. Do not use silicone lube if you are using silicone toys. The chemical added to keep silicone lube fluid will destroy the toy. Lube with spermicide can cause allergic reactions in many people, often realized as burning and itching. Lubes that have sugars added to them (j-lube, etc) can cause yeast infections in people with vaginas. Water-based lubes are generally safe to use in any situation.

Anal hooks can be a lot of fun but it should be remembered that they are a butt plug style toy, not something to bear weight. Too many people think that they are used to suspend the body. I can not even imagine the damage that would do to the body. I've seen tears caused by anal hooks after some tugging/pulling on them, never mind the forces involved in suspending the whole body.

Never insert anything into an anus that doesn't have some sort of base. Items that are cylindrical can get lost in the bowel and colon. Butt plugs and other ass toys have a flared base or a handle like an anal hook. This is so the body doesn't pull them into itself. Many embarrassing emergency room trips could have been avoided if people had followed this simple rule.

Any time the mouth comes in contact with the anus, you run the risk of some rather unpleasant consequences. Many people enjoy rimming/analingus but use a dental dam to do so. Others take the risk, making sure that they are freshly showered and as clean as possible. Hepatitis A and various bacteria can be spread through oral contact with fecal matter, so be aware.

Cock rings and chastity devices can cause problems if they are too small. A ring that seems the right size when flaccid can easily be too small when hard. Make sure the ring is suitably sized or has some flexibility to it, otherwise things can get rather painful - and not in a good way!

Photos and videos serve as a sexy reminder of the fun you had, but can also quickly turn into blackmail material. We are all familiar with the concept of revenge porn. Be very careful who you allow to photograph or video you naked or in sexual positions. You may want to ensure that your face is not in the frame (not so useful for those of us covered in custom tattoos).

Exhibitionism can be fun when done within the confines of a sex allowed play party or swing club. Doing sexual things in public where it's not allowed is a good way to get a sexual offender label that will follow you around for the rest of your life, possibly affecting your ability to obtain housing, jobs, etc. Think very carefully before you kink or fuck in public.

Permanent piercings of any sort should be done by a trained professional. Many are kink friendly and don't mind you involving a bit of kink in your appointment, within reason (and safety). This is not something you should attempt to do on your own, even if you've taken a play piercing class, the details of the two techniques are different.

Ravishment play can contain emotional landmines. Negotiate it thoroughly and have a safe word. Do not engage in this sort of play in public. The neighbours/bystanders won't know that it's a scene and may call the police. If outdors is a fantasy, look at joining one of the kinky camping events or doing so at a play party. Just don't forget to let the DM know what you're up to!

Ruined orgasms and post cum torture can bring up feelings of resentment, even when it's the bottom who asked for the activity. Tread carefully in this area until you know how you and your partner will react. Make sure you have a safe word or way to indicate that something isn't right if you need it.

Not all chastity devices are created equally. Some are meant for short-term wear and can cause health issues if worn long term. Even those intended for long-term wear must be removed and cleaned on occasion. How often will be determined by how easily you can clean with the device on.

Choosing Activities

We will be using the same basic method of choosing activities as we have before. However, instead of choosing 3-5 activities to try out, we will only be picking 1-2. Sexual taboo can be difficult to overcome and there can be a lot of emotional landmines hidden in our ideas towards sexuality.

It is important to take things slowly, both in exploring and in the activities themselves. Now, if 3 activities that you want to try seem like they work well together and create the flow you want, you can certainly try that. For instance, someone exploring anal play may want to engage in rimming (licking around the anus), fingering the anus, and anal sex with either a penis or dildo/strap-on. Those activities make sense, preparing the recipient by increasing arousal (hopefully).

Compatible activities rated 4/5 or higher:

Who will top? Who will bottom?

Compatible activities 3/5:

Who will top? Who will bottom?

What positions will the bottom be in?

Which activities are off the table (listed as 2/5 or lower)?

What safer sex precautions will you need to take?

What other preparations will you need to take (enemas, STI screening, etc)?

Planning Your Scene

As you can see, there are a number of potential pitfalls - and we haven't even talked about some of the intricacies of adding other people to your sex. As with any new activity, taking things slow and keeping the lines of communication open is vitally important.

I am a firm believer in having a safe word or signal at any point when resistance or ravishment is involved. You may find that you only want to use a safe word or signal the first few times. If you are worried that it will take away from the realism of the scene, try it once with a safe word. You can always do it again without one when you're more comfortable. I am a safety nut, so always want to have a way for my bottom to communicate any problems, but your risk tolerance may differ.

When exploring sexual taboos, adding one or two (or a category, such as our earlier example of anal play) at a time is the best approach. You don't want to overwhelm yourself or your partner, trying a dozen new things at once. It doesn't matter whether you're on the top or bottom, it can be a sensory and mental overload.

Jamie & Taylor's Sexual Taboo Negotiation

Jamie and Taylor decide that they want to explore chastity, as well as some edging to keep it interesting. They decide that the chastity will last for three days since Taylor usually masturbates or engages in sexual activity at least once a day. Jamie will have control over the number of times per day that Taylor is to edge, and the timing of it.

They decide that after the three days, the scene will end with a wild sex scene. Taylor must please Jamie to earn an orgasm, otherwise, the chastity will continue for an additional two days. Taylor thinks this will be easy, Jamie thinks Taylor will be begging for release after a day or two.

Their usual safe words will be in effect. In addition, if Jamie asks Taylor to edge when it is inappropriate (Taylor is at work, for example), Taylor does not have to comply immediately but will edge at the next reasonable opportunity.

Jamie also plans to send Taylor sexy messages to help with the edging and wants to engage in a little teasing. Jamie is allowed to masturbate and it is agreed that this information can be used to tease Taylor.

Since this is their first experiment with chastity, they will be using the honour system. If they enjoy it, they may consider a device. It is up to Taylor to abide by the agreement they have made, Jamie trusts that Taylor will be honest.

The Chastity Scene

Taylor and Jamie have a standing date every Friday night. With this in mind, they agree that they will meet for coffee after work Tuesday, at which point Taylor's chastity will begin. They are strangely nervous when they meet.

There is a sense of tension between the two, knowing that Taylor won't be allowed to self-pleasure unless it's for the purpose of edging for the rest of the week. Jamie is somewhat aroused by this prospect, unsure if it's the sexual nature of chastity or the power aspect that is more titillating.

Over the next few days, Jamie has Taylor edge a few times a day. They exchange sexy text messages frequently. They find that the denial of sexual activity brings the sexual urges and feelings that Taylor has into sharp focus.

By Thursday, Taylor is begging to be allowed to masturbate. Jamie says no, that it's only one more day. Taylor grudgingly agrees, sticking to the negotiated terms of this play is more important.

On Friday, Taylor can't wait to see Jamie. Work takes forever and it's hard to focus. When Jamie messages, requesting more edging, Taylor asks not to. Taylor doesn't think edging is possible, there is too much pent up sexual energy, an accident may occur. Jamie understands and says it's okay, wait until they are together.

When evening finally rolls around, Taylor is full of energy and determined to please Jamie. They haven't really defined what that means, so Taylor will just do all the things that Jamie loves and hope it works.

In the end, Taylor is allowed release.

What Can We Learn?

Even if something seems simple, like going without a sexual release for a few days, it isn't always. It's one thing to go without for a while and not think about it, it's another entirely to not be allowed to forget about your denial.

Like any sexual taboo, going slow is important. Taylor probably couldn't have lasted a moment longer. They may have been a bit too ambitious to start with, by adding in the edging and sexual teasing.

Taylor spoke up when a request seemed impossible. This is important to be able to do. It is better to say "I don't think I can do this" and allow your partner to make a decision - take the risk or forget the request. While this isn't such a big deal when it comes to edging, it could be something more serious.

Being able to tell your partner no in a respectful way is an essential skill to learn in BDSM and in life. Calmly explaining what the issue is, why you are concerned and what the possible outcomes could be is good communication. You can then make decisions based on all the information, rather than withholding and winging it.

Of course, learning that chastity is often a deeply sexual activity, despite outward appearances, is a valuable lesson. We often want what we are told we can't have.

Overcoming Sex Negative Programming

If you have been told all your life that sex and sexual activity is wrong, immoral, dirty, disgusting, or otherwise undesirable - except for procreation within a marriage - you may have a hard time dealing with exploring sexually.

There is no one way to overcome this programming. You may be able to work through it on your own, with the help of your partner, or you may need to sit down with a psychologist and figure things out.

You can find dedicated sexual therapists in most places, and they are generally knowledgeable about kink and BDSM. They are there to help you and not to judge. You may need to interview a few (go to a first session to see if you're a good match) before you find one that you click with. Don't give up, but also do your best to work through some stuff on your own.

Having a supportive partner will make many things easier. If they can help and encourage you in your sexual exploration, fantastic. They may also be struggling with the same sex negative programming. Couples therapy may be in order then.

Joining a community of sex-positive people can also help. You can see them enjoying their sexuality without guilt. You can see that it's normal. You can see people expressing their sexuality in different ways, even see those of us who aren't into sex but encourage others to explore and enjoy.

The community can also help with some of your feelings of guilt. If others can enjoy sexuality on their own terms and still be good, moral people, so can you. You can see them acting ethically towards others regarding sex and in general.

Depending on what you've been taught growing up, your personality and how deeply ingrained sex negativity is, this can take a while to overcome. Like anything, taking small steps and reflecting on your feelings as you go is important. If you jump in with both feet, you may suffer from a lot of guilt after, or it may be the right approach for you. You know yourself best and what is most likely to work.

25 Exploring Sexuality & Sexual Taboo: Aftercare and Scene Review

The world of sexual taboo can be littered with emotional landmines but it may also be incredibly rewarding for you. Depending on your approach to sexuality, your beliefs around sex, and those of your partner, this can be a very liberating area to explore.

Sexual Taboo Specific Aftercare

It is hard to say exactly what people may need after exploring this type of play - there is such variety in the play and in the people who are interested in trying it. Let's start with the physical.

If you explored anal play for the first time or took it a bit further than you're used to, you may be feeling a little sore. Don't worry, it's perfectly normal. You inserted things in a place that's only used to travel in the other direction. Some tenderness or soreness for a day or two is normal, pain is not.

You may also notice that you have a strong urge to have a bowel movement, again this is normal. When you do, your stool may be a little loose. This is partially because of the lube you've introduced. If you see small traces of blood, it's alright. Again, your body isn't used to this yet, so there may be micro tears, no matter how careful you were. If you see a large amount of blood, that is not normal and may need medical intervention.

The same rules apply if you experimented with fisting, unusual or large insertions. Some discomfort is normal, pain is not.

If you have engaged in forced orgasm play, you may be dehydrated, so be sure to drink plenty of water. It's probably wise to have a snack too!

If you've tried pumping (genitals or nipples), expect the area to be a little sore. You may even notice some bruising or discoloration. If the bruising bothers you, you may need to ease up a little next time until your body gets used to it. There is, of course, a point where if you use enough suction, you're going to bruise no matter what.

If you've experimented with non-monogamy, you may want to spend some time reconnecting with your primary partner. Have some quiet time, cuddle, touch each other and reassure the other that you had a good time. You may even want to go for round two.

If your partner seems off in any way, be open to talking about it, but don't press the issue. They could be dealing with feelings of sadness, guilt or shame that have nothing to do with you and everything to do with negative programming they had earlier in life. Reassure them that you still love them, that they aren't a bad person and that they have nothing to feel sad about. You made an adult choice and had some fun. No one was hurt, and you shared something intimate with others.

If the non-monogamy involved humiliation, like in cuckolding or cuckqueaning, you may need to reassure the bottom partner. Let them know that the relationship is still intact, that you won't be leaving them for the bull or another woman.

In a hotwifing situation, reassure her that you enjoyed watching her with others. Tell her she made you proud when she did something notable. Tell her what part you enjoyed the most (flip the genders if it's a guy being shared).

If none of the above applies, proceed to whatever aftercare you typically enjoy. Many people will have no guilt or negative feelings after non-monogamous play, so enjoy it if that's you.

Sexual Taboo Scene Review

As always, it is important to talk about the scene you did. You want to make sure you're on the same page before moving forward or repeating something that one of you didn't enjoy. Look out for partners who are going along with things because they feel obligated or like they will lose you if they admit it wasn't as much fun as they wanted it to be.

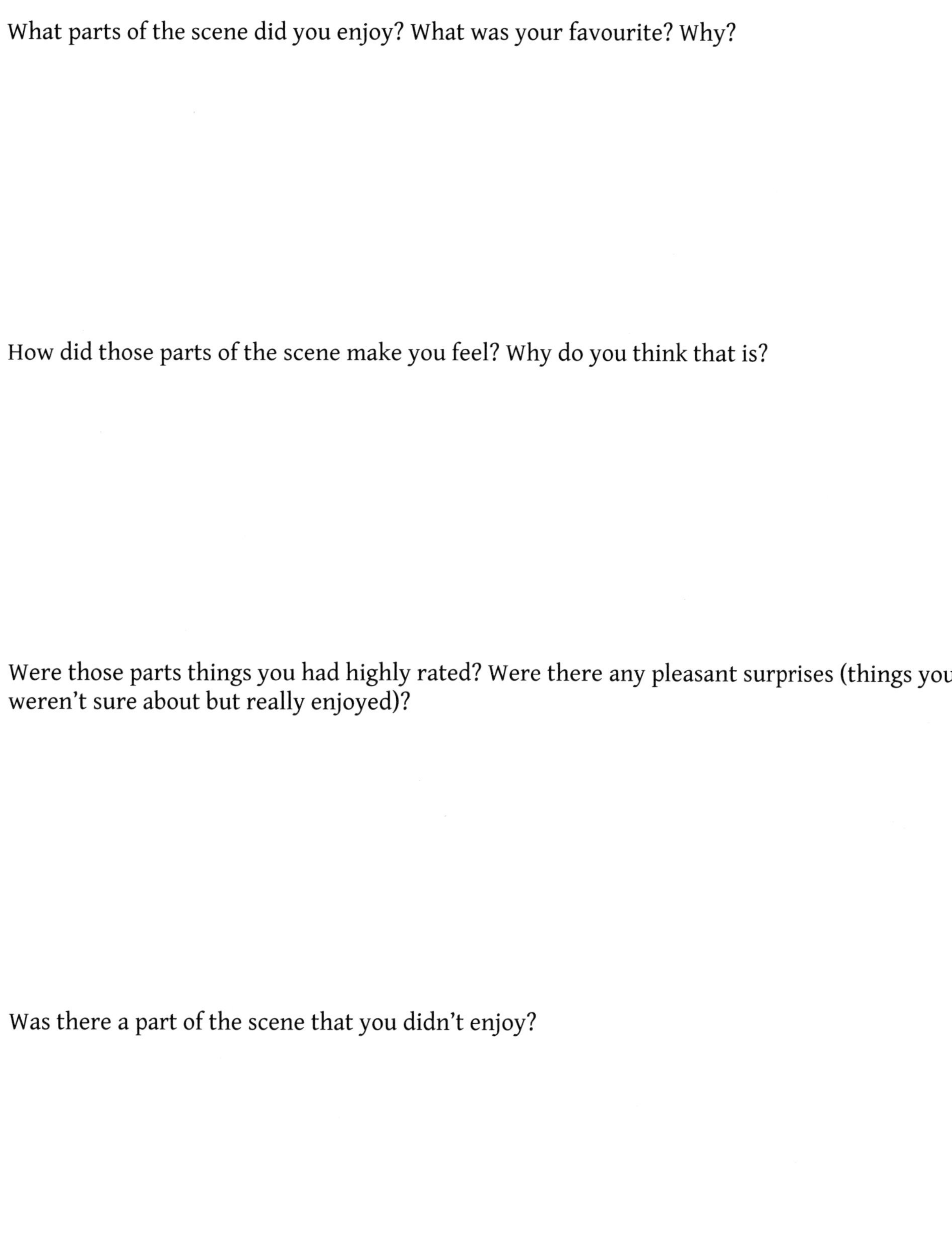

What parts of the scene did you enjoy? What was your favourite? Why?

How did those parts of the scene make you feel? Why do you think that is?

Were those parts things you had highly rated? Were there any pleasant surprises (things you weren't sure about but really enjoyed)?

Was there a part of the scene that you didn't enjoy?

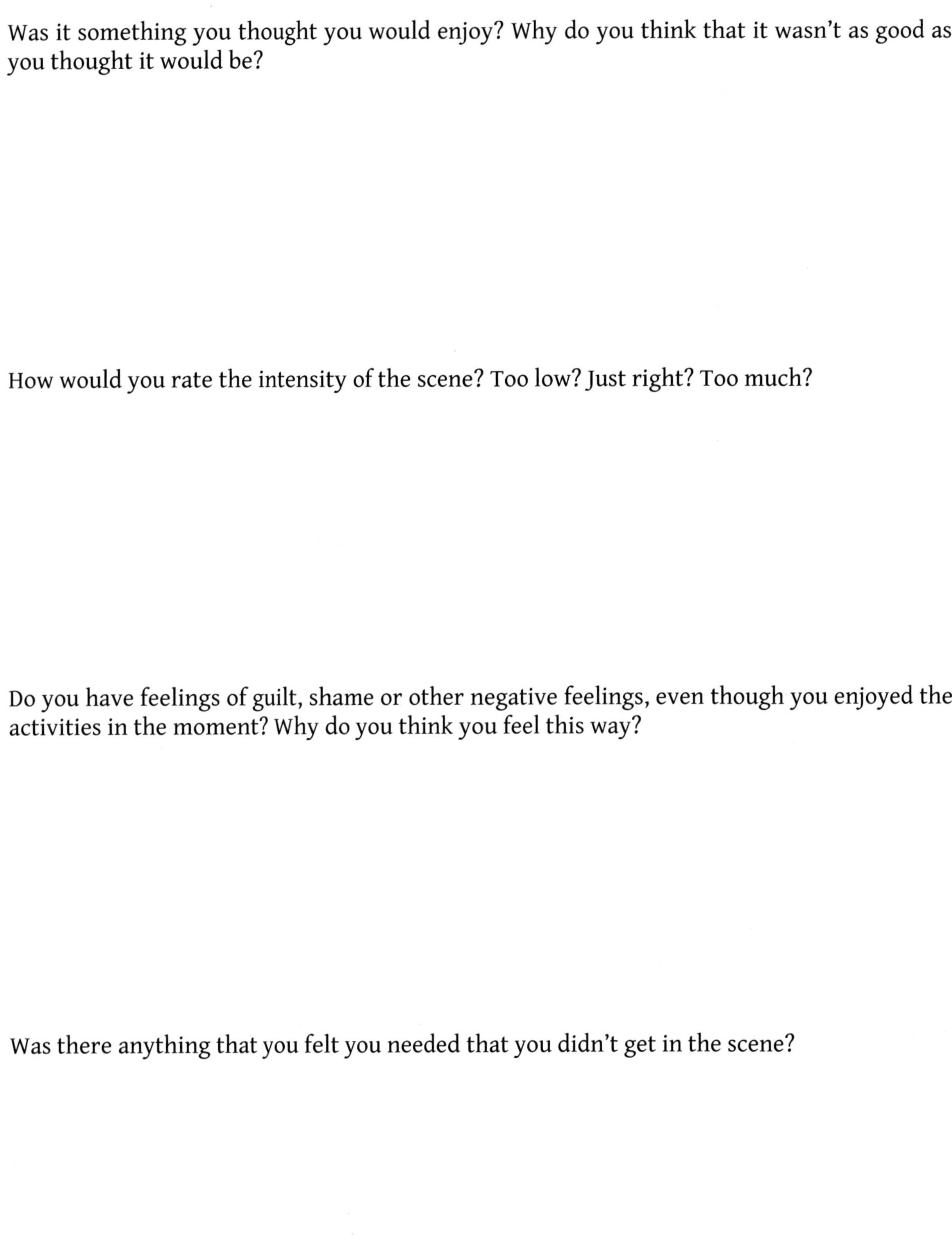

Was it something you thought you would enjoy? Why do you think that it wasn't as good as you thought it would be?

How would you rate the intensity of the scene? Too low? Just right? Too much?

Do you have feelings of guilt, shame or other negative feelings, even though you enjoyed the activities in the moment? Why do you think you feel this way?

Was there anything that you felt you needed that you didn't get in the scene?

How do you think the scene went overall?

Did you find that the aftercare was sufficient? Did you drop?

Name one thing you would change for next time and one thing you would like to keep the same.

26 Exploring Role Play: Checklist

Role play is what you make it. You can have it be a simple affair, with just your imaginations and acting ability to carry you through. You can invest in props and costumes to make things as realistic as possible. How you do it is up to you.

There are some role play scenarios that require more thorough negotiation and contain potential landmines - things which can trigger strong emotional reactions. I've marked those activities with a ⚐. You may not want those role play scenarios to be your first experience of this type of play, or you may want to jump right into the deep end. It's up to you. Just be aware that you should talk a lot before and after these scenes.

Of course, you may have your own emotional triggers that will mean a particular scenario could be a problem. Proceed with caution if you choose to engage in those.

How to Use the Checklist

You may find it easiest to photocopy this list or download it from my website at www.MsMorganThorne.com if you prefer to do it online or print it out yourself. Of course, you're more than welcome to fill out this one right here in the book if you want to keep things all in one place.

Both or all partners should fill out this checklist, to gauge interest in activities and so that they are aware of what the other(s) are interested in. If you have multiple partners, each pairing should fill out a checklist, as what you are willing to explore with one partner may be different than what you are willing to explore with another.

Make sure you indicate your experience, if any, with each activity. Again, this is the beginning of a conversation, not the whole thing. Don't be afraid to ask a person how they learned, whether they were a top or bottom for that activity, etc.

If an activity does not apply to you for whatever reason, simply ignore it or write in **N/A**. Use a **T** or **B** to indicate that you would be interested in topping or bottoming for an activity. If you're interested in doing both, simply write both letters in.

Rating scale for the checklist. Remember, if you haven't tried an activity, indicate your interest level in that activity. If you plan on having others involved directly in your play, indicate with an * which activities you would want to keep between you and your primary partner or the person you are filling this checklist out with.

- **NO** is a hard limit, something you are not interested in doing under any circumstances.
- **0** (zero) is a soft limit, something you aren't interested in doing, but may consider under specific circumstances and with specific negotiation.
- **1** (one) is something you aren't really interested in doing but will oblige if it's requested occasionally.
- **2** (two) is something that you're okay with doing but you don't really enjoy. You will do it if asked, to please your partner, or as a special reward.
- **3** (three) is something that you neither like nor dislike. You're up for it if your partner wants to, but it's not something you would miss if it didn't happen.
- **4** (four) is something you enjoy doing and wouldn't mind doing often.
- **5** (five) is something you really want to do, something you would like to do as often as possible.
- **?** is something you don't understand or are truly unsure about.

Always remember that these checklists are not written in stone. You can change your checklist whenever you like. If you try something and it's not nearly as much fun as you thought it would be, change it's rating. If you didn't think you would like something but have warmed up to the idea, change it's rating. Don't forge to let your partner know about the change. These checklists are a great way to keep track of things and for spurring conversations, but most of us don't check them before each time we play. I recommend using pencil to fill out your checklist so that you can change it whenever you need.

There are five blank spots at the end of each checklist. If there is something that fits this category that I haven't included, write it in! I've also done my best to keep the lists somewhat short, which means I've left out some of the more extreme activities. If you are interested in more extreme play, make sure you get educated on how to do it safely, including attending workshops and reading all you can on the subject.

Name: Date:

Role Play Activity	Experience Y/N	Rating NO, 1-5, ?	Top or Bottom
ABDL			
Age Play			
Age Play (Little)			
Age Play (Middle)			
Age Play (Big)			
Age Play (Adult Baby)			
Age Play (Parent/Child, Sister/Brother, etc)			
Age Play (Incest) ⚐			
Alien Abduction			
Alien Impregnation/Eggs			
Animal Play			
Animal Play (Horse)			
Animal Play (Dog)			
Animal Play (Pig)			
Babysitter Role Play			

Role Play Activity	Experience Y/N	Rating NO, 1-5, ?	Top or Bottom
Bimbofication			
Daddy/Mommy Dominant			
Damsel/Dude in Distress			
Diapers (Wearing)			
Diapers (Wetting)			
Diapers (Soiling)			
Doctor, Nurse, Patient			
Erotic Dancer/Entertainer			
Fantasy Abandonment ⚐			
Funishment Scenes			
Furry Play			
Incest Role Play ⚐			
Initiation Rites			
Interrogation Play ⚐			
Kidnapping Fantasy ⚐			
Maid Role Play			
Master/Mistress & Slave Role Play			

Role Play Activity	Experience Y/N	Rating NO, 1-5, ?	Top or Bottom
Nazi Role Play ⚐			
Online Role Play			
Pet Play			
Pet Play (Kitten)			
Pet Play (Puppy)			
Pony Play			
Prison Role Play			
Ravishment Play (Rape Play) ⚐			
Religious Role Play			
Ritual Play			
Satanic Ritual Scene			
School Role Play			
School Teacher			
School Student			
Sex for Money Fantasy ⚐			
Slave Role Play (Historical) ⚐			
Slave Role Play (Gor)			

Role Play Activity	Experience Y/N	Rating NO, 1-5, ?	Top or Bottom
Slave Role Play (Other)			
Stranger Role Play			
Wild West Role Play			

27 Exploring Role Play: Scene Creation and Ideas

Role play is such a common kink that even vanilla people get up to it sometimes. It can take many forms and you can take it as seriously as you like. Some people enjoy a simple costume or wig and some dialogue. Others will go to great lengths to achieve realism in their role play.

Many people use role play to explore fantasies that they would rather not actually engage in. A classic example is a couple who may want to sleep with other people but don't want to actually commit to sleeping with other people. They will role-play the scenario, pretending to be strangers. They meet, maybe at a regular bar, maybe at a swing club. They decide to have a one night stand or even an ongoing affair. Maybe they take turns being the sexy stranger, maybe it's only one of them.

I've even met people who have used the above scenario to try out a cuckold situation. The one pretended to be another person, they slept together and then the "cheating" spouse tells the "cuck" all about the affair. It's one way to test the waters.

Now, you will have to choose one scenario at a time, unless you can make things work together. For instance, someone interested in ABDL (adult baby, diaper lover) can incorporate that in with a babysitter roleplay but not a firefighter one (unless you get really creative).

Role Play Specific Safety Concerns

There isn't a lot to say here. Some of the "edgier" roleplays can be triggering for some people, especially if they are using this sort of play to work through past trauma. Having a safe word is always wise, especially in situations where you know there is a history.

Recognizing someone who is triggered can be difficult. They may go nonverbal but still be compliant. They may freak out. They could have any reaction in between or may show no outward signs of stress. Check in with your partner often if you are playing with a potentially triggering subject.

If you are playing with themes which could be triggering to others - like people watching at a play party - you should consider if it's really something you should do in that space. Authentic slave trade play, race play, play involving realistic firearms or police uniforms can all be upsetting to many people, often people of colour or other minority groups. Think about if your ability to play this way in public is worth making them feel unsafe. If you're planning that type of scene for a party, check with the host first as it may not be allowed, for the above reason.

If you are engaging in kidnapping or sex for money role plays, make sure that you do this away from the public eye. You don't want to have to explain these things to the police if someone sees you and you really don't want to have to hire a lawyer!

Compatible activities rated 4/5 or higher:

Who will top? Who will bottom?

Compatible activities 3/5:

Who will top? Who will bottom?

Will you be including activities from a different category of kink? If so what are they?

Who will top? Who will bottom?

Which activities are off the table (listed as 2/5 or lower)?

Planning Your Scene

This is one of the easier scenes to plan. You need to choose a scenario. Then you need to decide how much time and effort you want to dedicate to making it realistic. Do you have an old Halloween costume that would work? Items in your wardrobe?

By putting a bit of thought into your scenario, creating a backstory, even if it's just a few sentences, it will help when it comes time to enact it. You give your character motivation to do the things they're doing. It's like performing an improv play - you get a few key elements but you need to flesh it out and make it come alive.

If you're going to incorporate other BDSM elements and activities into the scene, what are they? Have you done them before? Make sure you have everything you need and try not to introduce too many new elements at once.

Does this scene require a safe word? Will there be resistance involved? Will coming out of character act like a safe word or signal?

Once you've decided these and the typical negotiation elements, you're pretty much ready to go.

Lead by Example

Rather than have Jamie and Taylor give us an example scene here, I'm going to relay an ongoing scenario I had with a charming gentleman. It wasn't what you would expect, but it was a lot of fun every time we got to do another addition to this scene.

He had a thing for naughty school girls. Not just any naughty school girls but really mean, Catholic school girls that would torture and shame him. He liked being the authority figure who fell from grace and had no choice but to do what the mean girl wanted. She was blackmailing him with humiliating and painful acts.

I would catch my teacher masturbating at school, vowing to tell the principal and the whole world if he didn't do exactly as I said. He was at my mercy, lusting after me even as I stomped all over him, figuratively and literally.

I tried to think of various items that I could use that were school related. There is the obvious items; rulers, yardsticks, etc. Office supplies are intriguing for torture. Elastic bands can be snapped against the skin of the nipples and genitals to great effect. Binder clips make wonderful clamps. A textbook will make a decent paddle, even without a handle. "Steal" some rope from gym class, or a wicked looking electrical contraption from the science lab (TENS or violet wand) and you have endless scene possibilities.

I also did simple things like having him crawl around. I would wear a chain around my waist that he knew turned into a leash and collar. I rode on his back like a sad little horse, making him carry me around the room or else I would stab my high heels in his thighs. I trampled him and hit him with my hands. We also incorporated a bit of verbal humiliation, but I'm not a huge fan of it, so it was limited. Something to note here, it was easier to include the verbal humiliation because I was playing a role and "not me".

Those are just a few ideas you can use for a number of scenes. Many of those things would work for a secretary/boss role play. The key here is imagination. Really get into the character, think the way they would think.

A Sample Scene

In the same vein as above, here is a sample scene for that scenario. It is probably similar to one of the many scenes I did along these lines since there were many.

A "school girl", complete with super short kilt and white (see-through) blouse walks into a classroom after school has let out, saying she forgot her phone/bag/homework. She catches her teacher jerking off at his desk. After an initial freak out, she calms down and has an evil thought.

He is begging her to forget what she saw, offering money or whatever she wants, just don't tell anyone. Whatever she wants...

She has a pretty sadistic streak, so she tells him that he will be her slave. To play with and do whatever she wants to do. If he doesn't, she will not only expose his jerking off but tell everyone he touched her here (pointing at an inappropriate place for a teacher to touch a student).

At first, she's excited but nervous. She doesn't really know what to do with her new slave. She makes him crawl around on the ground, kiss her shoes and tell her she's the smartest and prettiest girl in school.

In a moment of inspiration, she grabs the porn magazine that he was jerking off to, finding it's all BDSM and Femdom stuff. She laughs at him, asking if he's into this "sick shit". He's further humiliated. He berates him about his taste in porn, even though she also likes the images. She decides that she will recreate the picture he was jerking off to.

She sees a banana on his desk and figures it's the right shape...

She makes him crawl around on the floor with a banana sticking out of his ass, her laughing and insulting him the whole time. She teases him "I thought you liked this sick shit? Why isn't your little cock hard yet?" She then makes him jerk off in front of her, while she slings insults his way. When he begs to cum, she allows it but only if he cleans up the mess with his tongue. He agrees.

What We Can Learn

Aside from the fact that I'm pretty evil, we can see that you don't need anything fancy to do a great scene. All you really need is an imagination. This scene and the many like it that I did, didn't require much equipment. I could have done it in a dungeon or a living room. I sometimes brought some props into the scene, like the textbooks or elastics mentioned above. We sometimes used traditional dungeon toys when we wanted to mix it up a bit.

I will point out that if you are going to stick something like a banana in a person, put a condom over it first, just in case a piece breaks off or there are rough edges.

Are you ready to get creative with your own role play scenarios?

Feeling Silly

You're going to feel silly for the first few minutes of any role play. To get started, it's easier to leave the room - one of you or both - then come back in while you're in character. It will still feel strange for the first little bit, but if you're trying, it should fade quickly.

I've found the only times I really feel silly doing roleplay is when my partner didn't play along. It can be really awkward if they don't give you anything to go off of.

I say that, having played a female WWE style wrestler, multiple times, a spy who was interrogating the wrong person, a crazy doctor/nurse/surgeon/scientist more times than I can count, and many, many more. Imagine screaming "Tell me where the plans are!" in a terrible German accent at a man who is looking at you like you have two heads, then talk to me about feeling silly!

28 Exploring Role Play: Aftercare and Scene Review

The aftercare that you may need to do after a role play scene will heavily depend on the elements of the scene. Did you incorporate a lot of other BDSM play into the scene? Then take a look at those sections for tips on aftercare.

Was the subject matter of your roleplay emotionally taxing? Then you may need to support your partner or mutually support each other while you work through that. It is not unusual to cry a bit after a heavy scene that opens up old wounds or that engages you with disturbing elements of history. Don't worry about it, your partner will still respect you if you cry after playing out a tough scene.

It's hard to go into too much detail on aftercare because what one person needs can vary so much in this type of scenario. Read the other sections for specific advice and just go with what you feel you need.

Reviewing the Scene

After a few hours or days, sit down to talk about the scene. What went right and what didn't so you know for next time. If you felt silly throughout the whole scene, try to find out why.

Was your partner not into it? Were you not into it? Did you have a hard time connecting with your character? If any of those are the case, you may try a more scripted scenario. Start with a rough outline of where you want the scene to go, but leave lots of room for improvising. Don't start writing lines or anything. You may also need to put a bit more thought into the characters you're playing - if you have a bit more to work with, you may find your groove.

Don't give up after one or two bad role play scenes. Try different scenarios until something clicks. If you've tried a variety of scenes and characters, without it going well, maybe roleplay isn't for you. That's okay! There is a lot more to explore in the world of BDSM.
With that said, let's get to our typical questions about the scene:

What parts of the scene did you enjoy? What was your favourite? Why?

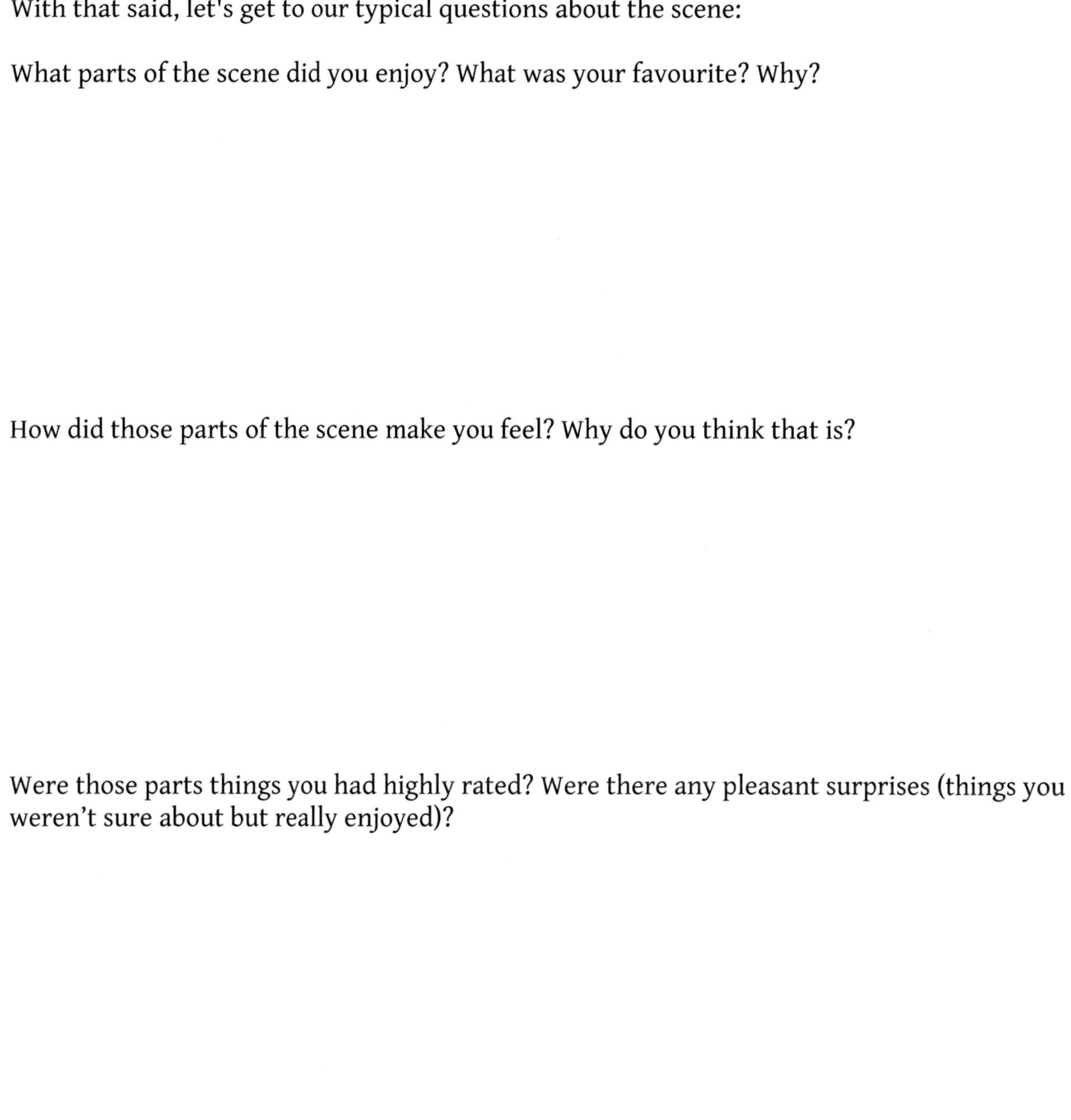

How did those parts of the scene make you feel? Why do you think that is?

Were those parts things you had highly rated? Were there any pleasant surprises (things you weren't sure about but really enjoyed)?

Was there a part of the scene that you didn't enjoy?

Was it something you thought you would enjoy? Why do you think that it wasn't as good as you thought it would be?

How would you rate the intensity of the scene? Too low? Just right? Too much?

Would you be interested in trying that activity again or would you prefer to leave it for a while (or permanently)?

Was there anything that you felt you needed that you didn't get in the scene?

How do you think the scene went overall?

Did you feel silly the whole time or just at the beginning? Why?

Is there another character or scenario that you would like to try? What is it?

Name one thing you would change for next time and one thing you would like to keep the same.

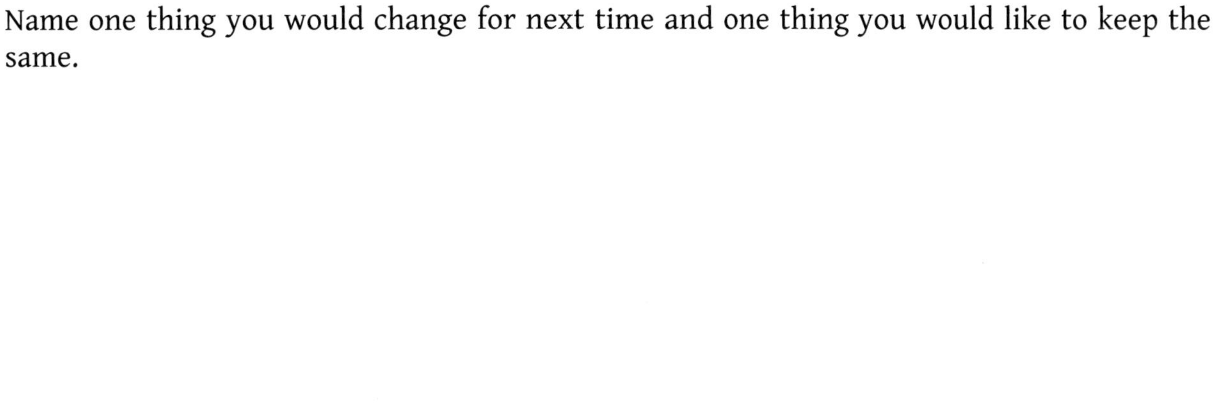

Feel free to add any questions that you think are important. Remember that BDSM isn't just a physical experience, it's a mental and emotional one too. Make sure you address all of these aspects when you have your scene review. Even though it may be hard, it is really important, to be honest with your partner, otherwise, they may end up doing things you don't enjoy inadvertently.

29 Exploring Humiliation Play: Situational vs Personal

Humiliation can fall into different categories, depending on how you want to look at it. I've divided it into situational and personal humiliation. Additional categories may include verbal, degradation, objectification, and public humiliation. For me, those are parts of the two categories above. Your approach may be different and that's totally okay.

When I talk about situational vs personal humiliation, it's the target that shifts. In situational, the person may be in a humiliating situation, either because they were "forced" into it or through their own poor choices. Personal humiliation is picking at an aspect of the person themselves, they may be unattractive, not very smart, or lacking in skills.

You can probably tell by my language above that I am far more comfortable with situational humiliation than I am with personal humiliation. For me, it's the difference between something I find amusing versus a personal limit.

Just because I'm not into something, doesn't mean it's not wildly popular as a kink. Humiliation, in general, is very popular. It seems to be popular across all gender identities, sexual orientations, etc fairly equally. It's not that common to see a kink that's enjoyed nearly equally between bottoms like that. I will specify bottoms because I see many male identified tops who enjoy giving humiliation, but fewer female identified ones who do.

It may be the type of humiliation or the specific requests that come in. Many male bottoms enjoy the "worthless worm" style humiliation they see in porn, while I know fewer female tops who enjoy it. I will say that the ones who do, seem to really enjoy it, so it's not all lost for humiliation fans seeking a toppy woman!

But Why?

If you're like me, you may not understand why humiliation is such a popular kink. Think of it as emotional masochism - just as people enjoy the physical sensation of pain, some enjoy the emotional pain that comes along with being degraded.

Through humiliation, the bottom can be stripped of their pride. They can be torn down so that only the core of who they are is left. A lot of humiliation play involves rebuilding the bottom at the end of the scene or the idea that the top uses it to break the bottom, to later mould them into who they want them to be.

Humiliation can also render the bottom helpless, similar to the feeling evoked by bondage. These feelings of helplessness and worthlessness allows them to pursue their fantasies without having to admit full responsibility for liking them. I don't mean that in a negative way, sometimes it's hard to admit that we like what we like. Who else would enjoy being used as a toilet, for example, other than a "worthless" person? (I don't believe that, but it's an example of the thought process.)

By breaking down the ego or even the sense of self, humiliation can help some people overcome sexual inhibitions. It's a way to be vulnerable to your partner so that you can share intimacy.

Humiliation is an intensely personal kink too. I can't tell you how to humiliate your partner. What I think would be humiliating, they may find boring, or way over the line. It is such a unique and individual kink that it's hard to learn if it doesn't come naturally.

Don't worry, I will give you a bunch of ideas to get your creative juices flowing and there's always the checklist to get you started.

Situational Humiliation

Humiliation by placing a person in embarrassing or degrading situations can be an easier pill to swallow for some tops. You aren't attacking who the person is, just kind of making fun of them for being in a bad spot. If your partner is into humiliation, this may be a good way to ease into it, but it may not be enough for some people or hit the right buttons.

Pet and animal play can sometimes fall into this category. Even if the human animal is treated as a cherished pet, they are still less than human. Of course, many pet and animal players don't find this to be humiliating at all, so your mileage may vary.

Requiring the bottom to ask permission for normal bodily functions may be humiliating for some. To be treated like a child who needs to ask permission for everything, even going to the bathroom, can be deeply humiliating. Simply talking about such personal matters with a partner may also be humiliating for some. To push it even further, make them leave the door open so you can see and hear if you choose. Forcing a person to use the bathroom in front of another can be incredibly embarrassing (or no big deal, you know your bottom best).

Covering the bottom in bodily fluids is considered by many to be humiliating. Covering them with cum, spit, or urine can hit all the right erotic humiliation buttons for some people, others need to push it further, being forced to consume said fluids.

Eating one's own fluids is another popular humiliation tactic. Adding an element of "force" is optional but fun.

Still, others will feel humiliation by being put on display. They may be stripped naked while the top is clothed or they may be required to wear a specific costume. They could be bound in a way that leaves them very exposed or used as an object. Serving sushi on naked people is a fetish in and of itself, tied in with turning people into objects.

Objectification can also include human furniture or posing as human art. It can be difficult to maintain a certain pose, be ignored and be unable to interact as a human.

Cuckolding and cuckqueaning, as discussed in the Exploring Sexuality and Sexual Taboo Section are types of situational and personal humiliation. Some activities will cross over between multiple types of humiliation.

Enemas can be a deeply humiliating experience, especially if the top wants to watch the bottom expel it. Some people have no problem urinating in front of others, but defecation is totally different. The sounds and smell can be very embarrassing, even for the most hardcore humiliation bottom.

For some men, cross-dressing can be a humiliating act. The fetish of forced feminization and sissy-hood seem to be rooted in misogyny, whether the person into it realizes it or not. Being embarrassed to be dressed as a woman does not sit well with a lot of people. There doesn't seem to be a corresponding kink for being humiliated by dressing like a man.

Personal Humiliation

Personal humiliation attacks the ego. It breaks down the person through insults and cutting remarks. Comments don't have to be true to be effective.

Calling names is both the easiest and hardest way to verbally humiliate a person. You need to know the words that humiliate without going too far. While most people will be okay with being called a bitch, cunt, asshole, jerk, pervert, sick, etc. many will object to things like fat or stupid, that attack core beliefs about themselves or bring up insecurities.

Find out what is okay and what is off limits before playing and expect to find a few emotional landmines along the way. Have a plan for how to deal with them when they happen. Your partner may not be in a state of mind to tell you how to help in the moment. Some will want reassurance, other will want to be left alone. You won't know until you talk about it or it happens.

Insulting their abilities is another common theme. They may be a lousy lover, an inadequate provider, or just generally useless. Find out what shakes them to the core.

Body image is another hot button that may work or work too well. Insults about the size of a person's penis are so common that there is a category of humiliation known as SPH or small penis humiliation. I'm unaware of a specific fetish for other body parts but I have played with one woman who loved to hear how stinky and smelly her pussy was (it wasn't). Humiliation may involve a bit of acting. Many of the people I've known into SPH had anything but small penises.

A good tactic for the beginner is to give the bottom a choice between two bad things (they can just be different words for the same thing too). "Are you stupid or inept?" makes them choose between two things no one wants to be. Make them pick one and say it out loud, really rubbing it in if you feel like it.

Intensely Personal

Once again, humiliation is intensely personal. You will need to communicate thoroughly with your partner to find out what they like and what their limits are.

We often forget that tops or dominants get to have limits too. In this case, it is brought into focus for some people. They may be able to beat a bottom bloody, but they feel guilty calling them names or being "mean" to them. If this is a limit for your partner, try to find what they would be comfortable trying.

Using myself as an example again, I enjoy putting people in embarrassing situations. I do not like insulting them. I can call a person a slut or slave because I don't see those things as being insulting. I could not tell a bottom that they were fat, ugly or stupid, I would feel terrible for weeks.

30 Exploring Humiliation Play: Checklist

Humiliation is such a personal thing. What humiliates one person is no big deal to another. It is almost impossible to classify any of these activities as being more complicated than another. I will leave it up to you to decide what is actually humiliating and what may be emotionally triggering.

How to Use this Checklist

You may find it easiest to photocopy this list or download it from my website at www.MsMorganThorne.com if you prefer to do it online or print it out yourself. Of course, you're more than welcome to fill out this one right here in the book if you want to keep things all in one place.

Both or all partners should fill out this checklist, to gauge interest in activities and so that they are aware of what the other(s) are interested in. If you have multiple partners, each pairing should fill out a checklist, as what you are willing to explore with one partner may be different than what you are willing to explore with another.

Make sure you indicate your experience, if any, with each activity. Again, this is the beginning of a conversation, not the whole thing. Don't be afraid to ask a person how they learned, whether they were a top or bottom for that activity, etc.

If an activity does not apply to you for whatever reason, simply ignore it or write in **N/A**.

Use a **T** or **B** to indicate that you would be interested in topping or bottoming for an activity. If you're interested in doing both, simply write both letters in.

Rating scale for the checklist. Remember, if you haven't tried an activity, indicate your interest level in that activity. If you plan on having others involved directly in your play, indicate with an * which activities you would want to keep between you and your primary partner or the person you are filling this checklist out with.

- **NO** is a hard limit, something you are not interested in doing under any circumstances.
- **0** (zero) is a soft limit, something you aren't interested in doing, but may consider under specific circumstances and with specific negotiation.
- 1 (one) is something you aren't really interested in doing but will oblige if it's requested occasionally.
- **2** (two) is something that you're okay with doing but you don't really enjoy. You will do it if asked, to please your partner, or as a special reward.
- **3** (three) is something that you neither like nor dislike. You're up for it if your partner wants to, but it's not something you would miss if it didn't happen.
- **4** (four) is something you enjoy doing and wouldn't mind doing often.
- **5** (five) is something you really want to do, something you would like to do as often as possible.
- **?** is something you don't understand or are truly unsure about.

Always remember that these checklists are not written in stone. You can change your checklist whenever you like. If you try something and it's not nearly as much fun as you thought it would be, change it's rating. If you didn't think you would like something but have warmed up to the idea, change it's rating. Don't forge to let your partner know about the change. These checklists are a great way to keep track of things and for spurring conversations, but most of us don't check them before each time we play. I recommend using pencil to fill out your checklist so that you can change it whenever you need.

There are ten blank spots at the end of this checklist, because humiliation is so personal. If there is something that fits this category that I haven't included, write it in! I've also done my best to keep the lists somewhat short, which means I've left out some of the more extreme activities. If you are interested in more extreme play, make sure you get educated on how to do it safely, including attending workshops and reading all you can on the subject.

Name: Date:

Humiliation Activity	Experience Y/N	Rating NO, 1-5, ?	Top or Bottom
Anal Plugs (Public, Under Clothes)			
Animal Play (pet, dog, horse, etc)			
Begging/Grovelling			
Bimbofication			
Blackmail			
Body Worship			
Burping			
Cuckold / Cuckquean			
Cum Eating			
Degradation			
Diapers			
Emasculation			
Enemas			
Exam (Physical)			
Face Slapping			

Humiliation Activity	Experience Y/N	Rating NO, 1-5, ?	Top or Bottom
Face Spitting			
Foot Humiliation			
Forced Bad Wetting			
Forced Pants Wetting			
Forced Masturbation			
Forced Nudity (Private)			
Forced Nudity (Public Sex Club/Dungeon)			
Forced Servitude			
Forced Cross Dressing			
Humiliation (Private)			
Humiliation (Public)			
Human Art			
Human Ashtray			
Human Furniture			
Human Toilet			
Inspection (Physical)			
Insults			

Humiliation Activity	Experience Y/N	Rating NO, 1-5, ?	Top or Bottom
Objectification			
Pig Play			
Phallic Gags			
Phallic Worship			
Poses (Exposure, Embarrassing, etc)			
Put on Display			
Removal of Privacy			
Sexual Humiliation			
Sexual Inadequacy Humiliation			
Shaving (Body Hair)			
Shaving (Head Hair)			
Shared Sexually			
Slut Training			
Small Penis Humiliation			
Spitting			
Verbal Humiliation (Private)			
Verbal Humiliation (Public)			

Humiliation Activity	Experience Y/N	Rating NO, 1-5, ?	Top or Bottom
Watching Bathroom Activities			

* Lots of blank spaces to fill in your own answers because humiliation is so personal!

31 Exploring Humiliation Play:

Scene Creation and Ideas

You can create a scene based on humiliation or use it as an element in a scene. It is flexible enough that you can use it in just about any scene you choose. When planning a scene that involves humiliation, you should decide if you will include other BDSM activities as well. Keep in mind that what one person finds humiliating, another won't care about and a third will have it as a hard limit. Communication is key here.

Humiliation Specific Safety Concerns

The big safety concern is mental and stumbling across emotional landmines that the bottom was unaware of. Keep in mind that many bottoms will keep going, even if they don't want to, as a way to try and please their top. This can be especially true in humiliation scenes.

The humiliation may shake their self-confidence so they are less likely to speak up. They may also start to believe what you are saying - that you really think they are worthless, just an object of sexual gratification and nothing else. This may cause them to endure in an attempt to be worth something, by making you happy.

Keep an eye out for a bottom that's in this state because of a hidden landmine. You may need to check in frequently in the beginning and anytime you are unsure if they are still enjoying the play. Use your judgment. You can always play harder next time, but you can't take it back if you go too far now.

Public humiliation can be tricky too. You may want to enjoy an audience but what effects will that have on you and your bottom?

Will someone you work with see you and think you're an asshole, passing you up for a promotion?

Will a family member see your bottom and stage an intervention to get them away from you, who they think is an abusive partner?

Will you run afoul of the law, ending up with a sexual offender designation because of consensual kink done in the wrong place?

Keep in mind that the general public has not consented to be a part of your scene. You should not be shoving your humiliation fetish on them. If you want to indulge in some public embarrassment, do so at a play party, where people have consented to see kink in action. It's much safer and more ethical.

Compatible activities rated 4/5 or higher:

Who will top? Who will bottom?

Compatible activities 3/5:

Who will top? Who will bottom?

Are there any keywords, phrases, or actions that provide a good humiliation for you? What are they?

Are there any keywords, phrases, or actions which are taking things too far? What are they?

Which activities are off the table (listed as 2/5 or lower)?

Will you combine other activities with humiliation? If so, what activities?

Planning Your Scene

You should spend more time talking about this type of scene in the beginning than many other types of scenes. You will need to find out what is okay, how far is too far and what is a hard limit.

It's also advisable to have some sort of safe word or signal during the scene, just in case. Your partner may enjoy denying or trying to defend themselves against your insults, so you need a way to communicate when they've hit the limit.

Picking a place to do your scene is important. If you want an audience, you may have to wait for the right play party. If you're doing a private scene, you can plan for whenever you want.

Make sure you prepare the other elements of your scene if you're including them. Bondage can heighten humiliation if tied in an exposed manner. Spanking can enhance a scene where the bottom is being treated like a child. You may need to lighten up on some elements because of increased emotional sensitivity.

Jamie and Taylor's Negotiation

Jamie and Taylor want to indulge in a public scene. There is a party this weekend at a local dungeon. They begin planning an elaborate scene.

Jamie wants to include some bondage so that Taylor can't escape the public humiliation. They agree to rope bondage. Taylor will be bound naked during the scene. After the initial play, Jamie will place a sign around Taylor's neck, inviting others to spit on or pour drinks on Taylor.

To make that happen, they need to bring a tarp to protect the dungeon floor as well as some towels to soak up any drinks. They also make sure that the dungeon has a shower facility, so Taylor can shower after the scene.

They agree that Jamie will engage in name calling and verbal humiliation, making Taylor feel worthless and small.

They want to keep things short, as it's their first time playing with these themes. The first part will only last a few minutes, and the part where other people can join in will last for 10 minutes unless Taylor gives the safe signal before that. Jamie will pretend to ignore the situation, but won't go far and will really be watching closely for signs of distress.

The Humiliation Scene

When they arrive at the dungeon for the party, Jamie goes to speak with the DM on duty, to explain the plan for the humiliation scene. The DM approves the scene and makes suggestions as to where would be the best place to tie Taylor up. It is also suggested that they do the scene earlier in the evening or closer to closing time when there won't be such a big crowd that could block Jamie's view when monitoring.

Jamie also shares the safe signal with the DM, so that there are two sets of eyes on Taylor during the scene.

Jamie and Taylor chat nervously, trying to decide the best time to get started. They decide to watch some of the other guests play a bit, then start their own scene.

When the time comes, Jamie begins to bind Taylor in a compromising position. Jamie starts with muttering insults quietly, slowly growing louder. Jamie is surprised at how hard it is to say these things to a loved partner. There are some pangs of guilt, but Jamie remembers that Taylor really wanted this.

Taylor seems to be having a lot of fun, making eye contact with other guests, almost inviting them to watch. Part of the fun is having an audience. Taylor gets more excited as Jamie's insults get louder. At this rate, other guests will be able to hear them soon.

Jamie places the sign around Taylor's neck and promptly dumps a large glass of ice water all over Taylor. The ice collects in Taylor's lap, very cold against warm genitals. Some of the guests giggle at the scene. For good measure, Jamie spits in Taylor's face and half yells an insult. Taylor is thrilled, but Jamie feels guilty again.

As the guests read the sign, some of them decide to join in. They are making sure that Taylor is covered in a steady stream of spit and various drinks. Some even smear a bit of food from the snack table on Taylor. Jamie is surprised at how watching this is causing anger. Taylor seems very happy, so Jamie tries to play along.

When the agreed upon time is up, Jamie releases Taylor, who is bouncing around and excited. They move to where the showers are to get Taylor cleaned up. Jamie tried to hide the conflicted feelings but Taylor notices.

What Can We Learn?

Probably the most important lesson here is that tops have limits too. Sometimes, those limits aren't what they're willing to do, but what they're willing to allow to happen to their bottoms. Jamie was getting upset watching Taylor being humiliated and treated badly (in a consensual way) by others. It didn't matter that Taylor was enjoying it, it still felt like an insult to Jamie and triggered an urge to protect Taylor from the "abuse".

Humiliation, especially public humiliation, can be a hard pill to swallow for some people. If you're into it and your partner is hesitant, take it slow and move at their comfort level.

Often humiliation is a kink requested by and driven by bottoms. It's something they want, so they ask for it. Not all tops are able to deliver, so it is something that should be talked about early, like any other kink that is important to you.

32 Exploring Humiliation Play:

Aftercare and Scene Review

Humiliation scenes may need more aftercare than other types of scenes. There is the idea that a top will break down a bottom during the scene and part of aftercare is rebuilding their self-confidence. At the very least, many people will need a hug and some reassurance after an intense scene like this.

Humiliation Specific Aftercare

Reassurance is probably going to be the big thing for humiliation. Making sure the bottom knows it's all just play and assuring the top that the bottom still loves/likes them. The more intense the humiliation, the more reassurance needed.

Personally, I find that after scenes that involve humiliation, I need a hug from my bottom, to reassure me that we are still friends or lovers. Some tops may need this sort of things after an intense pain scene, others will need it with humiliation.

Of course, if there are physical aspects involved, the bottom should be checked for injuries and to make sure they are physically okay too.

I am a firm believer that unless there are some pretty extenuating circumstances, that we should look after the bottom's well-being first, then attend to our needs as tops. It's part of the responsibility we take on. Think about being a team leader in any field. You attend to the needs of your staff/players/people first, then your own.

Cuddling, hugging and just generally getting back to the way the relationship was before the scene will make those involved feel better if they are feeling unsure of themselves.

If both the top and bottom enjoyed the play equally, they may not require much aftercare at all. They may want to engage in sexual activity or enjoy some connective touch.

A check-in a few days after the scene is always a good idea, but it is especially important after psychological play. Sometimes drop or other negative effects of play can take a few days to manifest. This can happen to both the top and bottom. Try to touch base after a day or two and make sure you're both doing okay.

Reviewing the Scene

Once you've had a few days to process, sit down and talk about the good, bad and ugly of the scene you shared. Maybe the scene went too far, maybe it didn't go far enough. This is where you need to speak up about what you want and need from a scene if it didn't go down the way you wanted it to.

It's easy for scene reviews to feel accusatory to a top. Keep that in mind if you ever have a scene that didn't work the way you hoped it would. Be gentle in your criticisms, as tops should be gentle with bottoms who didn't meet their unspoken expectations.

What parts of the scene did you enjoy? What was your favourite? Why?

How did those parts of the scene make you feel? Why do you think that is?

Were those parts things you had highly rated? Were there any pleasant surprises (things you weren't sure about but really enjoyed)?

Was there a part of the scene that you didn't enjoy?

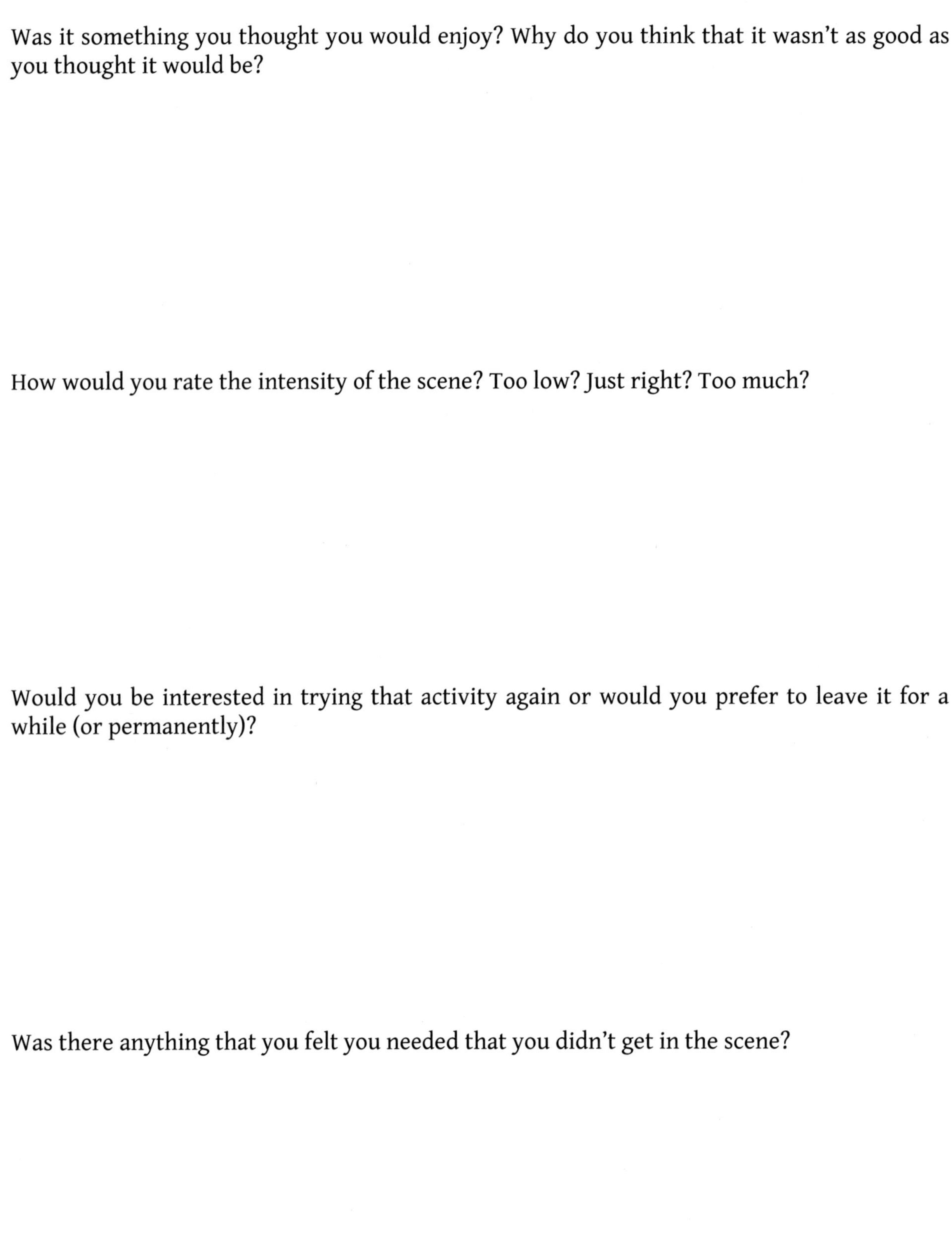

Was it something you thought you would enjoy? Why do you think that it wasn't as good as you thought it would be?

How would you rate the intensity of the scene? Too low? Just right? Too much?

Would you be interested in trying that activity again or would you prefer to leave it for a while (or permanently)?

Was there anything that you felt you needed that you didn't get in the scene?

How do you think the scene went overall?

Did you find that the aftercare was sufficient? Did you drop?

Name one thing you would change for next time and one thing you would like to keep the same.

Feel free to add any questions that you think are important. Remember that BDSM isn't just a physical experience, it's a mental and emotional one too - especially when it comes to humiliation. Make sure you address all of these aspects when you have your scene review. Even though it may be hard, it is really important, to be honest with your partner, otherwise, they may end up doing things you don't enjoy inadvertently.

33 EXPLORING PROTOCOL AND POWER EXCHANGE: POWER EXCHANGE RELATIONSHIPS AND RULES

Throughout most of this book, we've talked about play, the fun side of BDSM. What we haven't touched on very much is the power exchange side, the D/s. Domination and submission are, in their hearts, about authority. Who has it and who doesn't. Who leads and who follows.

If you would like to incorporate some power exchange elements into your relationship, it's best to take things slowly (I'm sure you're shocked, just shocked that I give this advice!). Start with one or two areas of control or authority, then add to them. Only engage in areas you are comfortable with and remember that you can renegotiate at any time (although for some people, that may mean ending the relationship).

Bedroom Only D/s

Many people start out and stick with bedroom only D/s. The name itself is a bit of a misnomer as this temporary assumption of authority can apply to any room or any time that the people involved agree to. It earned the name bedroom only because the area of authority is generally sexual.

You can negotiate that the dominant partner has control over your shared sex life, making the decisions about where, when, how often, and what is involved in your sexual encounters. Partners still need to negotiate the terms of the power exchange, what is included and what isn't. Everyone is allowed to have hard limits and should have a say in when/if their soft limits are pushed.

24/7

A lot of people misunderstand what 24/7 D/s is. They think that it's all gimp masks and leather corsets all day long. Nothing can be further from the truth. 24/7 D/s refers to a continuous power exchange, where one partner is always in control and holds the authority in the areas negotiated. A dominant in this style of relationship may be responsible for making decisions regarding the couple's sex life, social life, vacations, pets, etc. They may have put limits on finances and jobs, which remain egalitarian, the same as any other relationship.

Total Power Exchange

In a total power exchange relationship, the dominant holds all the authority, over every aspect of the shared life that the couple has. The dominant is responsible for making the decisions regarding work, leisure time, where the couple lives, etc. The submissive has agreed to follow the dominant's lead in every aspect.

Who Holds the Power?

It's commonly said that the submissive holds all the power because they have the ability to use a safeword or walk away from the relationship. It's true that they can do these things. It's also true that the dominant can do those things as well. Both people hold power equally in this instance. Dominants aren't automatons who can't help but dominate until someone puts a limit on their desires.

They are, however, people who have agreed to take on the authority and responsibility that goes along with that in a relationship. They exchange this for the obedience of the submissive, who agrees to follow the dominant's lead.

Questions to Ask Yourself

If you are thinking about entering into a D/s relationship, no matter what side of the slash you're on, you should be asking yourself some questions.

- What do dominance and submission mean to you?
- What are you hoping to get out of a power exchange relationship?
- What feelings or emotions do you expect a power exchange will deliver?
- How much control are you willing to take/give up?
- Do you want a bedroom only dynamic or 24/7?
- What does your ideal relationship look like?
- What are some concrete steps you can take to get there?
- What does my perfect dominant/submissive look like? What qualities do they have?
- What are my dreams and plans for the future?
    - Am I willing to give any of those up for the right partner?

- What do I have to give in a power exchange relationship (experience, skills, anything really)
- Do I want to be in my D/s role at all times, just sometimes, only during play?
- What does authority look like to me?
- Is there a difference between dating partner/spouse and D/s partner?
- Do I want a romantic relationship, love?
- Do I want both D/s and a romantic relationship with the same person?

Archetypes in D/s

Archetypes can be helpful in determining a theme of a relationship. They give us a well-known idea that we can relate to, seeing ourselves in one of the characters, so that we can build on that foundation to create a real relationship. These are the cultural icons and myths that evoke a strong narrative just by being named. I can say Mother & Child and you will have an image in your mind, including characteristics for each person.

I will start with the archetype that speaks to me the most, although it's can often get mashed up with a few others.

Lady/Lord and Knight

The Lady/Lord and knight is a classic BDSM archetype. It is seen more in F/m relationships, but there is no reason it can't apply to folks of any gender. It is still my preferred archetype when I am in relationships with other women.

This archetype has the dominant in the role of Lady/Lord. The one in command, the one who gives the orders. They are also the one who must care for and take responsibility for the knight. The submissive has the role of knight, powerful in their own right but recognizing the natural leadership or advantages of lending that strength to the Lady/Lord.

In this archetype, both partners are powerful, working together for mutual benefit. One leads, the other follows. This archetype also lends itself to higher protocol relationships as well, as many of these archetypes are formal relationships.

For me, I just love the thought of having command/control over a powerful person. I want a submissive who submits because they want to, because they see qualities in me that are worthy of their submission.

Similar archetypes could be Captain and First Mate, Priestess/Priest and Handmaiden/Monk.

Teacher and Student

The teacher-student relationship is one of teaching and making the submissive a better person. That's not to say there isn't strict discipline and rules to follow, there are. They help mould and shape the submissive into the person the dominant knows they can be.

Relationships based on this archetype tend to have an age gap component. Often the submissive recognizes that they need a stern hand to help guide them and keep them on track while the work to become the best version of themselves. They may need someone to apply discipline where they lack the ability to regulate themselves.

Similar archetypes could be: Trainer/Animal, Head-Mistress/Master/Ward

Parent and Child

This archetype is very similar to the Teacher/Student one but has more of an emphasis on nurturing and caring. The dominant is still trying to guide the submissive to a better version of themselves but may be more of a parental figure rather than a more aloof educator.

Corrupter and Virgin

This archetype has some elements of teaching and training the submissive partner but with more focus on corrupting their innocence. Here, the corrupter can shock and horrify (in a happy, consensual way) the virgin, using their innocence against them. The best part is that the virgin can simply wake up the next day and be totally innocent again, ready for the corrupter to work their evil magic...

Similar archetypes can include: Predator/Prey

King/Queen and Servant

An archetype that may lend well to service-based relationships, the King or Queen is the ruler, while the Servant does what is needed to ensure that their life runs smoothly and they have everything they need. The Servant may not have a glamorous position, but it is an essential one.

The King/Queen may be a benevolent ruler or cruel, torturing the help.

Hero and Sidekick

The Sidekick is usually pretty awesome on their own but they must bow to the authority of the Hero, who runs the show. These two work together to achieve their aims, combining skills in ways that may be unconventional but always get the job done.

Villain and Victim

The villain takes great pleasure in making life painful for the victim. This could be through physical or emotional sadism. It could be by making too many demands and pushing the victim as far as they can go. The villain is not above using CNC and resistance style BDSM to get their way.

There are many more archetypes that you can use for inspiration. Find one that speaks to you and use it to cement your ideas about what you want in a power exchange relationship. These are a handy base to build off of, giving each participant a general idea of their role so that you can sit down together and better define those roles.

Key Values When Starting A D/s Relationship

As I have been preaching throughout the book so far, open and honest communication is probably the most important thing when entering into any type of relationship but especially a D/s one. Remember, one person will be trusting the other to make important decisions, hopefully with their best interests at heart. Another person will be trusting that their partner will follow through on their agreements.

Integrity is also important, following through and delivering on the agreements you made. If you can't live up to your commitments sometimes, it's understandable. When it happens all the time, it shows that the person is lacking in integrity and needs to embrace the concept of open and honest communication.

Trust is essential to any sort of power exchange relationship. Trust is built slowly, over time. Each promise kept, each commitment followed through, each hard conversation had. If a submissive cannot trust the dominant, how will they give authority to this person? They will be second-guessing the whole time, afraid to really let go. If the dominant cannot trust the submissive, how will they give commands if they don't know they will be completed, or make rules that won't be followed. It's a lot of energy to invest in a partner who tells you they don't care by breaking the trust.

It may not always seem like it on the surface, but mutual respect is so important to successful D/s relationships. A dominant must respect their submissive enough to make the best decisions possible for them. A submissive must respect their dominant enough to obey and support them in making those decisions.

First Steps into Power Exchange

Taking your first steps into a power exchange relationship can be difficult. It's best to select one area of your mutual lives that the dominant will be in charge of first. For many people, it's their sex lives.

The dominant gets to make all the decisions regarding sexual encounters. When they happen, with whom they happen, how often, what is done, etc. This must all be done within the boundaries that they both have set.

If this is enjoyable for both, feels good and natural, then they can expand the authority. If the dominant breaches trust by pushing limits inappropriately or flat out ignoring them, then it's time to reexamine the relationship.

The dominant may fumble in the beginning, especially if they are new to making decisions for two. The submissive should do their best to support them, offer advice when appropriate, and do their best to follow the rules.

Slowly expand the realm of influence that the dominant has until you're both comfortable and happy with the amount of power exchange. For some people, it will start and stop at the bedroom. For others, they will be on the way to TPE in no time.

Creating Rules

Many new dominants rush into making rules, either because they think they should have a list of 100 rules for their new submissive or because said submissive has been pressuring them for rules.

The problem with this haphazard approach to rule-making is that you probably don't actually care about any of the rules you've made. If you don't care about them, how do you expect the submissive to? Do you really want to spend all your time keeping track of and enforcing rules you don't care about?

Rules should have a purpose. There should be a reason for each rule you make. So before you decide on a rule, ask yourself what purpose does it serve?

Is it something to help the submissive? To give them structure, to help them in school or work?

Is it something to help the dominant? To make their life easier or to take some stress or pressure off of them?

Is it something to make the household run smoothly? Whether it's a shared household or two separate ones?

Is it something to make the relationship run smoothly?

Is it something that you both find arousing or sexy?

All of these are valid reasons for rules, and I'm sure there are many other good reasons that I haven't listed too. Decide what is most important to you at this time. Craft a rule that is simple yet unambiguous. It can be something as simple as "send a text before you go to bed each night" or it can be something that requires more detail, like instructions on making meals each night, complete with specific recipes

When you are first making rules, only add one or two at a time. Try to keep the total number of rules reasonable. You don't need 128 slave rules that end up being repetitive and contradictory. Rules should be simple to follow and there should be a list for reference. Write your list in pencil or use a shared document file where you can make changes or additions.

Remember, rules are supposed to enhance the relationship. If they aren't serving that function, why have them at all? It may take some time to find the specific rules which work for you, so don't get discouraged.

34 EXPLORING PROTOCOL & POWER EXCHANGE: CREATING PROTOCOLS FOR YOUR RELATIONSHIP

Protocol is used by many different people in the kink world. It's a way of ritualizing the rules of your relationship and adding a nice reminder of the power exchange during a normal day. If they don't appeal to you, don't worry! You don't have to use them if you don't want to.

BDSM protocols can take on many different forms. There are day to day protocols, small acts of submission or devotion that reinforce a regular power exchange dynamic, and scene protocols or play protocols that govern behaviour while playing or out in the kink community. Which you use will partially depend on your relationship - does your D/s extend outside of the bedroom?

What is a Protocol?

Protocols are rules or behaviours that reinforce the power exchange dynamic through the use of repetitive and ritualized actions or words. Protocols are intended to make real the power the dominant has over the submissive, to put it in tangible, physical terms. They may be practised at certain times during the day when certain events happen or all the time.

Protocols are generally very individual, each relationship will work out their own set if they choose to use them. Most of the time you probably won't even see them happening - they're just a part of day to day life. These types of protocol can be acted out in front of family, in vanilla public, or pretty much anywhere. This can be as simple as sitting down to a meal where the submissive should not eat until the dominant has taken the first bite.

Of course, there are times where we do want the protocol to be obvious because it enhances play or our relationship. These protocols usually only happen within a very specific context and would look out of place if it happened outside of that context. These protocols can be things which are done in private, such as a submissive waiting by the door, on their knees, to greet the dominant when they arrive home.

There are some protocols that fall between the two categories above, where it's obvious that it's a BDSM thing, but totally normal among kinky people. Sometimes these protocols are so comfortable that we might slip up and enact one in public, leading to a few looks. A perfect example of this one is the use of honorifics, calling the dominant "sir" or "ma'am". You can excuse it as southern American manners, but it will still get a few looks from the vanillas!

Finally, you may have heard of high protocols or high protocol parties. This simply refers to parties or other events where there are strict house rules that govern the behaviour of the guests. This can range from submissives not being allowed to sit on furniture to the ways that dominants and submissives may speak with each other and interact. High protocol parties can be a lot of fun to attend, just make sure you read the rules first and that they sit well with you. You wouldn't want to show up to a party with your very shy submissive only to find out that it's a clothed dominant, naked submissive party!

It is important to remember that there are no set protocols for the BDSM community as a whole. Each event, each group, each couple will have their own set of protocols (or not). Usually, if a group observes formal protocols, they will be clearly posted and new people will be directed to them.

The only real "universal protocols" in BDSM involve obtaining consent before doing anything, not touching that which does not belong to you (including people), and understanding that a chosen title or role does not elevate one or subjugate another. Dominants are not in charge of every submissive, all submissives aren't in service to every dominant. The only time this changes is if you choose to attend an event which has clearly stated rules which override these basic ones. Of course, it's always wise to be polite to others, to conduct yourself with dignity and discretion in public, and to be honest with those around you.

Types of Protocol

Verbal protocols refer to any rules that govern speech. Using honorifics, being differential, etc. Verbal protocols can be anything you want them to be, including don't speak unless spoken to and no talking back.

Dress or clothing protocols govern, well, clothing. What the submissive may where and when are described by this set of rules. Will they be nude at home, at parties, or wear a special uniform?

Sexual protocols set out the dominant's control over the submissive's sexual activities. Is permission needed to masturbate? To orgasm?

Daily task protocols are the rules that apply to day to day activities. Asking permission to use the bathroom, how much social media time is allowed, etc.

Social protocols govern social interactions within kink friendly communities. Is eye contact permitted from submissive to dominant? Are there rules of the party that need to be followed?

There can be protocols for any area of life where the dominant and submissive have agreed to enter into a power exchange. The protocols reinforce those rules and keep the power imbalance fresh in the mind. Don't forget, you don't live your whole life in kink friendly spaces. You will need to make allowances so that protocols can be followed while interacting in the vanilla world or they will likely be ignored. It's one thing to be nude at home. Leaving the house, it's illegal to be nude (also, I live in Canada). Even within the home, what happens when a delivery person arrives? Friends who have a "nude at home" rule also have a bathrobe beside the door, just for those sorts of occasions.

Some example protocols for inspiration;

- Always using an honorific for the dominant in private or kink spaces
  - Using a specific name for the dominant/submissive that vanilla people wouldn't notice but means something to you.
  - A nickname
  - Using the person's full name, rather than a shortened version of it
- Submissive referring to themselves in third person (be careful, this annoys a lot of people) "this slave would like to..."
- The dominant opens all doors, car doors, etc for the submissive. Submissive is to wait until the door is opened for them to proceed
- The submissive opens doors for the dominant. Better not keep them waiting!
- The dominant enters and exits a room first
- The submissive waits to be acknowledged before speaking
- Eye contact restrictions, submissive must keep their head lower than the dominant's head, etc.
- Submissive kneeling when greeting the dominant
- Submissive kneeling when presenting a drink, food, anything they've been asked to fetch
- Submissive sitting on the floor, rather than the furniture
  - Submissive always sitting at the dominant's feet
- Walking a pace or two behind the dominant
  - Walking on a certain side of the dominant
- Submissive carries toy bag
  - Submissive carries all bags
- Submissive makes sure that the dominant is served food or drink first

    - Waiting for the dominant to begin eating before starting
    - Standing until the dominant is seated
- Submissive is nude when possible
- Submissive lights the dominant's cigarette or cigar (or refills their vape?)
- Submissive fetches drinks and snacks
- Submissive does not leave the room without the dominant's permission
- Capitalizing all written references to the dominant, not capitalizing written references to the submissive, including names. W/we or O/our as examples (again, this one annoys others, known as slashy speak)

Which Protocols Work for You?

You can try out different styles and types of protocols, to see what works best for your relationship. Do you and your partner prefer strict adherence to a long list of rules? Are you more relaxed, only making the rules that are absolutely needed? Rules and protocols should be introduced slowly and have a grace period for learning and testing.

If you're new to the idea of protocols, you may want to try one out for a week then decide if you want to keep it. If you do, great. Write it down where it's accessible by both (all) partners. If you decide it isn't working or it's just too much work, forget about it and try something different. The idea here is that the submissive should be able to reasonably learn and follow the protocol you both decide on, without a lot of micromanaging from the dominant (unless, of course, you enjoy micromanaging).

Try out different types of protocols. Ones that you use day to day, ones that you use during playtime or at kink events and ones that you use in private. The lines can shift between private and kink community acceptable protocols, a lot of it will depend on your boundaries and comfort level.

It is important to remember that protocols are negotiated and agreed on by those who are using them. You can't expect other people to know or respect your protocol. This is often a point of contention when a dominant makes a rule that no one is to speak to the submissive without the dominant's permission. In this case, anyone wanting to talk to the submissive, friends, people at a party, etc. need to ask the dominant first. This can be viewed as imposing their dynamic on others. Some people may feel upset by this, especially if they already have a friendship with the submissive and suddenly have to start asking permission.

If you do decide to use protocols in your play or relationships, make sure you aren't imposing them on others. It's a good way to annoy people in the kink community and you will likely get called out for it if you try that sort of thing in the vanilla world - either by vanillas concerned for your partner's safety, or kinksters who don't want to be outed by association.

A quick tip on creating protocols that are easier to remember and follow; make them positive. A protocol ideally talks about what should be done, the way the dominant expects it to be. Imagine being handed a list of 25 things you couldn't do. I bet it would feel a lot more restrictive and smothering than a list of 25 things that should be done this way. Or 25 things you should do.

It's the difference between "the submissive may not go to the bathroom without permission" and "when possible, the submissive will ask permission to use the bathroom". "The submissive is not allowed to wear undergarments" is negative, where "the submissive will dress in a way the dominant finds pleasing" is a more positive approach.

You also need to decide how much detail goes into each protocol. I could have the rule "the submissive will dress in a way that is pleasing" and leave it at that. I would expect my submissive would pay attention to when I compliment their dress, or point out clothing that I like on them. I would then expect them to dress according to my expressed likes.

That might work wonderfully for some submissives and leave others completely lost. For a different submissive, I might have to detail that I prefer black jeans rather than blue, fitted with a boot cut. Black biker style boots. I prefer a fitted, black tank top or band t-shirt. In cold weather I prefer the leather jacket, but if the cold will be an issue, wear the parka. I may need to go into even more detail, letting them know what I like and don't like in their wardrobe.

For the submissive who prefers open ended rules that require interpretation, this would be miserable. For a submissive who prefers clear and concise requests, with a great deal of detail, so nothing is left to chance, this approach would be ideal. You will need to figure out which style works best in your relationship.

What Level of Protocol?

High protocol is great for a party. A somewhat complicated set of rules that covers social interactions, often clothing, who can sit where etc can be a lot of fun for an evening but it's a lot of work to do it all the time.

Maybe it's because I'm a low protocol dominant, but the idea of keeping track of all those rules, enforcing them and living by them seems pretty miserable to me. Usually, by the time the party is over and it's time to go home, I've had enough high protocol living to do me for a while.

Most people find themselves between low and medium protocol if they have a 24/7 style dynamic. For people who are bedroom only, they may enjoy adopting the formalities of a higher protocol dynamic for when they play. As with just about any other aspect of BDSM, do what works for you!

35 EXPLORING POWER EXCHANGE AND PROTOCOL: CHECKLIST

I have always said that activities are not dominant or submissive. There are some activities, however, that help to reinforce power disparity for many people. You won't often see a person who has power beg. It's rare to see a person who has given up authority doling out punishments. It can happen, but it's rare.

In this section, we will look at various forms of power exchange as well as some protocols that can help reinforce that dynamic. I have indicated the activities and dynamics that take a lot of negotiation and trust with a O symbol. If you're interested in those dynamics, do your research and take things slowly. Talk more than you think you need to, negotiate as thoroughly as you can and make sure you set aside times to come together as equals to check in.

How to Use this Checklist

You may find it easiest to photocopy this list or download it from my website at www.MsMorganThorne.com if you prefer to do it online or print it out yourself. Of course, you're more than welcome to fill out this one right here in the book if you want to keep things all in one place.

Both or all partners should fill out this checklist, to gauge interest in activities and so that they are aware of what the other(s) are interested in. If you have multiple partners, each pairing should fill out a checklist, as what you are willing to explore with one partner may be different than what you are willing to explore with another.

Make sure you indicate your experience, if any, with each activity. Again, this is the beginning of a conversation, not the whole thing. Don't be afraid to ask a person how they learned, whether they were a top or bottom for that activity, etc.

If an activity does not apply to you for whatever reason, simply ignore it or write in **N/A**.

Use a **T** or **B** to indicate that you would be interested in topping or bottoming for an activity. If you're interested in doing both, simply write both letters in.

Rating scale for the checklist. Remember, if you haven't tried an activity, indicate your interest level in that activity. If you plan on having others involved directly in your play, indicate with an * which activities you would want to keep between you and your primary partner or the person you are filling this checklist out with.

- **NO** is a hard limit, something you are not interested in doing under any circumstances.
- **0** (zero) is a soft limit, something you aren't interested in doing, but may consider under specific circumstances and with specific negotiation.
- 1 (one) is something you aren't really interested in doing but will oblige if it's requested occasionally.
- **2** (two) is something that you're okay with doing but you don't really enjoy. You will do it if asked, to please your partner, or as a special reward.
- **3** (three) is something that you neither like nor dislike. You're up for it if your partner wants to, but it's not something you would miss if it didn't happen.
- **4** (four) is something you enjoy doing and wouldn't mind doing often.
- **5** (five) is something you really want to do, something you would like to do as often as possible.
- **?** is something you don't understand or are truly unsure about.

Always remember that these checklists are not written in stone. You can change your checklist whenever you like. If you try something and it's not nearly as much fun as you thought it would be, change it's rating. If you didn't think you would like something but have warmed up to the idea, change it's rating. Don't forge to let your partner know about the change. These checklists are a great way to keep track of things and for spurring conversations, but most of us don't check them before each time we play. I recommend using pencil to fill out your checklist so that you can change it whenever you need.

There are blank spots at the end of each checklist. If there is something that fits this category that I haven't included, write it in! I've also done my best to keep the lists somewhat short, which means I've left out some of the more extreme activities. If you are interested in more extreme play, make sure you get educated on how to do it safely, including attending workshops and reading all you can on the subject.

Power Exchange or Protocol Activity	Experience Y/N	Rating NO, 1-5, ?	Top or Bottom
24 Hours a Day/7 Days a Week			
Authority (Holds)			
Authority (Gives Up)			
Bathroom Use Control			
Bedroom Only Control			
Begging			
Behaviour Restrictions			
Body Modification (Ownership)			
Body Worship			
Chastity			
Chauffeur			
Collar (Private)			
Collar (Public)			
Collar (Permanent)			
Consensual Non Consent			
Crawling			
Cuckold/Cuckquean			

Power Exchange or Protocol Activity	Experience Y/N	Rating NO, 1-5, ?	Top or Bottom
Day to Day Control ⚐			
Discipline			
Domestic Servitude			
Dominant/Submissive			
Examination (Physical)			
Exercise Requirements			
Eye Contact Restrictions			
Following Orders			
Harems (Serving with Others) ⚐			
Honorifics			
Housework/Chores			
Genuflecting			
Kneeling			
Lectures for Corrections			
Loaned to Others for Service			
Loaned to Others for Sex ⚐			
Master/Mistress/Slave ⚐			

Power Exchange or Protocol Activity	Experience Y/N	Rating NO, 1-5, ?	Top or Bottom
Micromanaging			
Micromanaging (Clothing)			
Micromanaging (Food)			
Mono/Poly Arrangement ⚐			
Obedience			
Orgasm Control			
Owner/Property ⚐			
Protocols			
Protocols (High) ⚐			
Punishment Dynamic ⚐			
Reprimands			
Ritual			
Rules			
Service			
Service (Boot Blacking)			
Service (Tea Service)			
Service (Sexual)			

Power Exchange or Protocol Activity	Experience Y/N	Rating NO, 1-5, ?	Top or Bottom
Service Submissive			
Serving Others			
Sexual Activity Control (Timing, Where, How Long, etc)			
Slave Auctions			
Slave Positions			
Speech Restrictions			
Tasks			
Tattoo/Branding as Sign of Ownership ⚐			
Total Power Exchange ⚐			
Training			
Wearing Symbolic Jewellery			

36 EXPLORING POWER EXCHANGE AND PROTOCOL: SCENE CREATION AND IDEAS

You have a few options for exploring power exchange and protocols. You can follow the same steps as we have before, filling out a checklist, determining compatibility, trying it out and doing a review. You can also sit down and negotiate some of the term and rules of a more ongoing power exchange.

If you are interested in creating rules and protocols, please refer to the previous two chapters, which should contain enough information to get you started. It's an activity that will take putting your heads together and getting creative.

If, on the other hand, you like the pattern we've established so far, let's take a look at how these elements can come together for a scene.

Power Exchange and Protocol Specific Safety Concerns

Some of these may not be safety concerns exactly, but things that could come up that you may not think of. For instance, if you're into the idea of bathroom control, what happens if you're not together? Does the submissive get to make their own decisions about when to use the bathroom? Are they expected to message the dominant to get permission? What if the dominant is in a work meeting or on the subway and can't answer the message? How long must the submissive wait before they may use the bathroom without permission?

Obviously, activities like body modification and specifically branding hold their own risks. Always go to a professional to have these services performed. I know some kinksters who think they can create and execute their own strike brands. I have never seen one that turned out well. I have seen more than a few that have become infected (burns are much more likely to become infected). Professionals in the body modification industry rarely use strike brands because they don't give good results. Electrocautery is the accepted method for branding humans, and it should be done by a professional. Don't worry, if you really want to be involved, there is a lot of aftercare required to form a good scar from the brand, and that's done at home.

If you are going to create exercise requirements for your submissive, make sure you know what you're doing. If you don't workout yourself, pay a visit to a doctor and a personal trainer. Figure out what your goals are (weight loss, health, fitness, etc) and they will be able to advise you on an appropriate regimen.

Eye contact restrictions can be useful in some scenes, but I find that it takes away a fair bit of the non-verbal communication that I have with a submissive. Often, they will bow their heads to avoid accidental eye contact or turn their heads away. Now, not only can I not see their eyes, I can't easily see facial expressions. You could also easily mistake discomfort for trying to avoid eye contact and miss an important signal that not everything is okay.

Slave auctions are fun but misunderstood. Before anyone gets too excited, there is not a place you can go and buy a slave literally. Slave auctions are usually done for a charity or BDSM club to raise money. People will volunteer themselves to be auctioned off, usually for a specific service (house cleaning, cooking, car washing, etc) and their friends will bid on them. Half of the time, it's their partner who outbids everyone else, if they have a partner. It's not a place where you can buy a girl/boyfriend.

Training is a kink. There is no official "submissive training" that is universal. Get that idea out of your head right now. Training is simply teaching the submissive how the individual dominant they are in a relationship with likes things done. For instance, the first thing I teach a submissive is how I like my tea. I drink a lot of tea each day (I don't drink coffee), and I like it a certain way. Universal training would not be able to teach a submissive this essential skill (for me), and if you took on a submissive that I've trained, I hope you like orange pekoe tea with a splash of milk and stevia.

Preparing Your Scene

As usual, answer the following questions. You will be selecting a few items to add to a scene with other BDSM activities.

Compatible activities rated 4/5 or higher:

Who will top? Who will bottom?

Compatible activities 3/5:

Who will top? Who will bottom?

Will you be including activities from a different category of kink? If so what are they?

Who will top? Who will bottom?

Which activities are off the table (listed as 2/5 or lower)?

Jamie & Taylor's Rules

Jamie and Taylor decide that they will implement some rules for use during play. They've had some time to experiment a lot more and it's looking like Taylor is quite the masochistic player. Jamie is always a bit nervous about going too far, so they've determined a method to make them both happy.

They will implement some play rules that Taylor can break to prolong or increase the severity of the scene. The play rules are typical of people into funishment style play and knowing that Taylor can "accidentally" earn more funishment eases Jamie's conscious.

The play rules they've decided to implement are:

1. Submissive will assume a funishment position and do their best not to move, even if no actual bondage is in place.
2. Submissive is allowed to moan, yell and make as much noise as they like but they may not talk back to the dominant.
3. Submissive will count the current strike and then say "Thank-you. I deserve another" after each strike during funishment. After the final strike, the submissive will say "Thank-you. I have learned my lesson"
4. Failure to adhere to these rules will result in the dominant starting over at the beginning of the funishment.

These simple rules will be easy to keep track of, add a bit of formality to some of the play scenes that they do and give Taylor the chance to rack up a lot of extra funishment if they're in the mood.

The Funishment Scene with Play Rules

Jamie and Taylor get set up for their play scene. They decide to do a school style role play where Taylor is the naughty student. They have a few paddles to choose from as well as a new flogger. Jamie has been practising with the flogger and is ready to use it on Taylor for the first time.

They begin with Taylor bending over the bed, legs slightly apart, ass in the air. Jamie says that there will be a short funishment with the flogger, followed by 50 paddle strokes. Every time Taylor breaks a rule, the counter on those 50 will reset, even if the mistake is made on the last stroke.

With the rules laid out, Jamie starts with the flogger. The flogger is a good warm-up tool because Jamie is just doing light circles and figure eights with it. Jamie's aim is not good enough with hard strikes to use those on a person yet.

After warming up with the flogger, Jamie grabs the first paddle. Jamie strikes Taylor and Taylor says "One. Thank-you I deserve another". This continues until the 25th stroke when Taylor is silent. Jamie waits a moment and then informs Taylor that the counter is reset to 0. Jamie switches the paddle for a more intense one and starts again.

This cycle repeats itself a few times before Taylor makes it to 50 strikes without "forgetting" to count or talking back.

What Can We Learn?

Play rules are a great opportunity to get feedback on a scene as well as encourage a top that may be worried about going too far or accidentally hurting their bottom. By creating rules that are just for fun, no one is upset if they're broken. Rules are created to serve a purpose, as we discussed earlier. In this case, it's to ensure that both Jamie and Taylor get what they need from play without guilt.

It also gives the couple a chance to role play some power exchange and decides if they want to enter into a genuine power exchange situation. A far cry from genuine power exchange, it is one method to try it on for a short while and consider if they want to negotiate some bedroom only authority transfer.

37 EXPLORING POWER EXCHANGE AND PROTOCOL: AFTERCARE AND SCENE REVIEW

Aftercare will depend on what type of activities that you did during the scene. If you did impact, look for any bruising or injuries and apply first aid. If you included an activity where the bottom needs reassurance, provide it. If your aftercare ritual is cuddling up with a glass of wine then go for it. You should be used to general aftercare at this point.

Scene Review

In this scene review, we will look at the same questions that we have for other activities, but we really want to focus on the new elements of this scene. This will depend on what sort of elements you decided to incorporate into the scene. Power exchange? Play protocols? Real Protocols?

Use these questions to figure out if your protocols need tweaking. You will notice that some of the questions are about how things felt. Sometimes, it's easier to describe how a thing felt rather than if it worked. How do we know it worked if we don't know how it was supposed to make us feel? By incorporating how you want to feel into any element of BDSM, we can tap into that part of us that is more instinctual. It can also help us have more satisfying kink scenes.

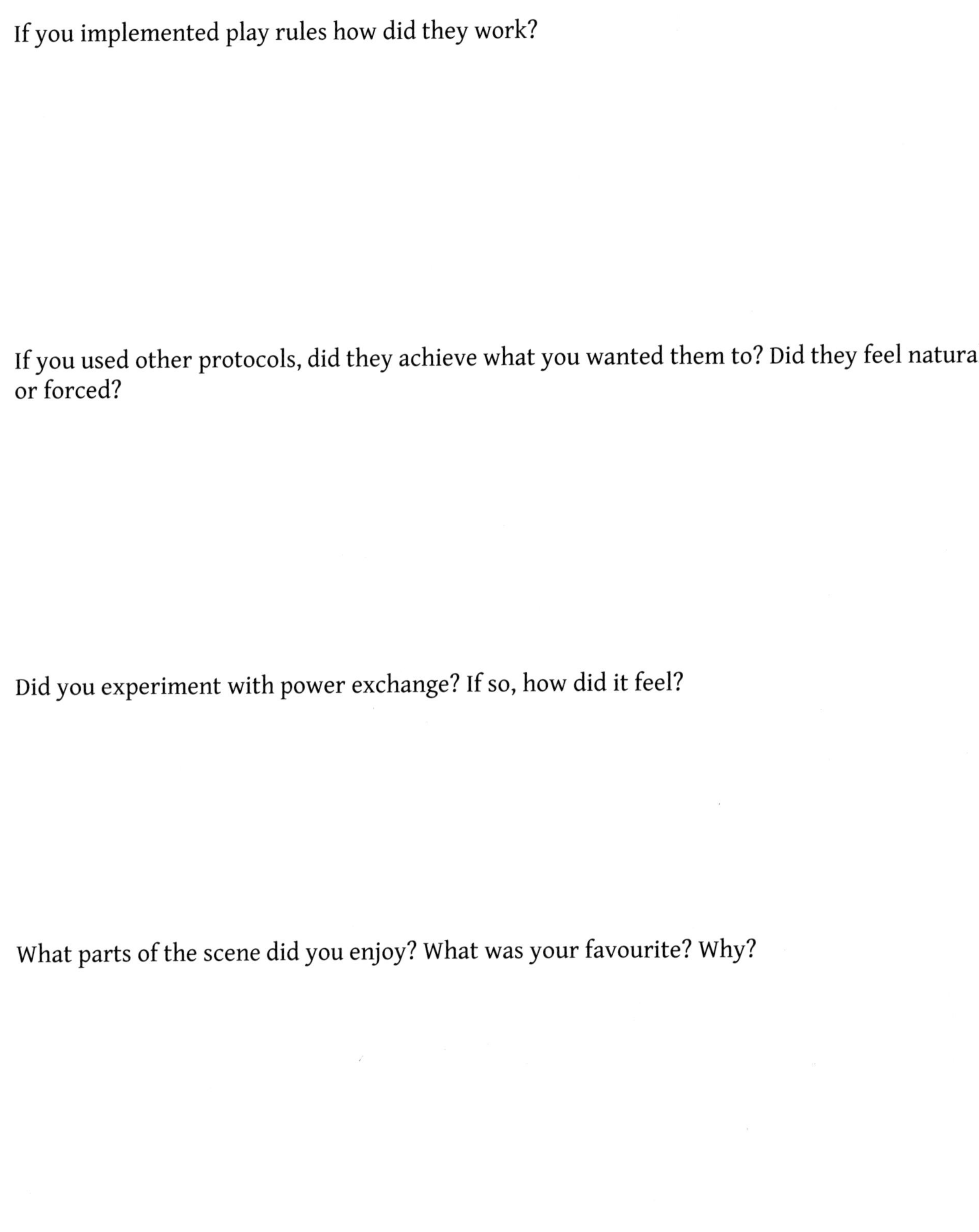

If you implemented play rules how did they work?

If you used other protocols, did they achieve what you wanted them to? Did they feel natural or forced?

Did you experiment with power exchange? If so, how did it feel?

What parts of the scene did you enjoy? What was your favourite? Why?

How did those parts of the scene make you feel? Why do you think that is?

Were those parts things you had highly rated? Were there any pleasant surprises (things you weren't sure about but really enjoyed)?

Was there a part of the scene that you didn't enjoy?

Was it something you thought you would enjoy? Why do you think that it wasn't as good as you thought it would be?

How would you rate the intensity of the scene? Too low? Just right? Too much?

Would you be interested in trying that activity again or would you prefer to leave it for a while (or permanently)?

Was there anything that you felt you needed that you didn't get in the scene?

How do you think the scene went overall?

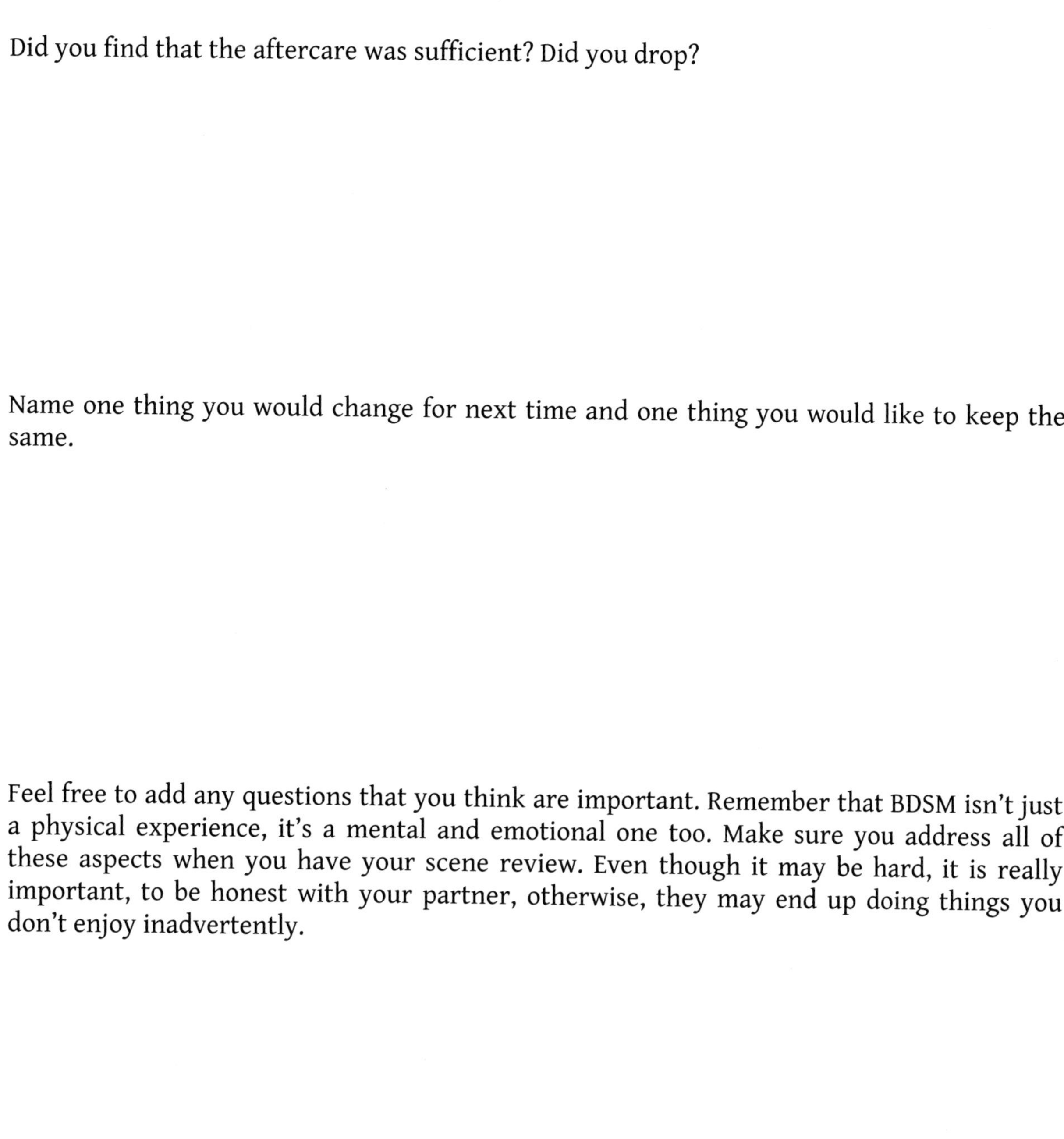

Did you find that the aftercare was sufficient? Did you drop?

Name one thing you would change for next time and one thing you would like to keep the same.

Feel free to add any questions that you think are important. Remember that BDSM isn't just a physical experience, it's a mental and emotional one too. Make sure you address all of these aspects when you have your scene review. Even though it may be hard, it is really important, to be honest with your partner, otherwise, they may end up doing things you don't enjoy inadvertently.

38 EXPLORING TABOO & EDGE PLAY: NOT FOR THE FAINT OF HEART

Taboo and "edge" play is not for the faint of heart. It probably doesn't have much of a place in a book for people new to kink. I'm including it because I find it impossible to talk only about the lighter side of BDSM when I know the dark secrets that are just a click away. You're going to find this stuff. It's all over the internet. At least if I include it here, I can say my piece.

Taboo Play

Taboo play are things that are a bit edgy and a bit offensive (okay, a lot offensive, sometimes). This category of play includes things like race play (using racial slurs and stereotypes during scenes). Those were one of the few scenes I would always turn down when they were requested for professional sessions. I could not bring myself to use those words, even at the request of a client.

Having said that, I do enjoy some taboo play. My skills when it comes to medical play combined with my enjoyment of consensual sadism has led to many WW2 inspired medical scenes, sans racial elements. I've engaged in "dark pet play" with a former partner, the combining of pet play and sexual elements.

If either of those things made you feel just a little off, you can see why it's called taboo play.

If taboo is something you would like to explore, tread carefully. It is important not to fetishize people because we have kinks. It can be a hard line to walk, engaging in this type of play while still respecting the humanity of your partner. It's also part of why there is an attraction to it.

The taboo nature of some things makes them erotic and attractive to some people. Walk that line carefully and err on the side of caution if you're worried about hurting others.

If you want to do this sort of play at public parties, you should always check with the organizer first. Some types of play will not be allowed. Some shouldn't be done because of the potential effects on other people there. I know the rule at parties is "if you see something you don't like, walk away" but there are some things that are too hard to ignore. You don't want to be the person everyone is talking about for crossing lines, do you?

We won't be doing the typical scene creation because I don't want you to do this stuff, at least not yet. Get a good, solid grounding in BDSM first. Explore all the exciting things that are now available to you. Look for things that you think are hot that aren't included on any of the lists here. I've left out a lot!

Later on, when you're ready, you can take a look back at this section. You can think about the things listed here and decide if you want to try them out. If you do, I urge you to get appropriate in-person training. I tour around a lot, maybe you can even attend one of my classes.

Edge Play

Edge play covers things which are dangerous. More dangerous than the typical BDSM activities. For instance, choking can cause brain damage or death. That's pretty dangerous compared to a spanking.

There are items on this list, like CBT, that are dangerous if done incorrectly but with some education, it can be much safer. The key is getting that education. I don't have space in this book to cover the world of genitorture here (one day, though!). The activities marked with a book should be things you can find classes on in your community. If they interest you, get out and take a class or two. Watch some videos online. Read up on them.

Edgier Edge Play

I would be lying to you if I said I didn't enjoy at least half of what's on this list. I've been around in the BDSM scene for more than 20 years now. I've also had an education in healthcare, worked in the body modification industry (and been a regular customer over the years). I've taken classes and learned how to do these things in the safest manner possible. Some of them are still deadly. Some of them are things I would never do because they are too dangerous (don't worry, I will let you know which ones those are).

Over the last 10 years or so, the attitudes towards edge play have shifted. It now seems like kink has become a competition, where everyone has to do the most extreme thing, even if they have no idea what they're doing.

I've seen skin tear because of improperly placed flesh hooks. I've seen needles fly out of a bottom and prick a few audience members because someone thought they knew what they were doing but really didn't. I've seen bottoms harmed because of pride and ignorance.

I'm not saying this to scare you off of the BDSM community. For the most part, it's a wonderful place full of amazing people and lots of resources for learning. Like all people, kinksters can get full of themselves. They can overestimate their skills. Learn from those people, learn to stay humble and not repeat their mistakes.

It used to be that edge players were the dirty little secret of the kink world. We were put in the back playrooms and kept away from the vanillas, in case we scared them away. Now, we are put on stages to perform for screaming crowds at fetish nights. Times change.

If you want to explore the world of edge play, learn from experienced and knowledgeable people.

39 EXPLORING TABOO & EDGE PLAY: CHECKLIST

There are items on this list that will probably horrify you. There may be a few that turn you on or catch your eye in some way. Some of these things you may recoil at initially, but find that with time the idea becomes more appealing. All of those are valid reactions.

The very nature of this list means that pretty much all of these activities aren't really suited for beginners. It's here to show you where you can go, if you choose. It's also here because there are always those people whose number one fantasy is something very taboo.

I've left off many things from this list. Feel free to add to it as you see fit. There is a whole perverted world out there and a million kinks you could try. I've tried to find a bit of middle ground, to give you a hint of what may be available for those who want it and trying not to scare off the new people! It's a fine line.

Like anything else, some of these things are more dangerous than others. Since we already said there isn't anything that's super beginner friendly, I've gone right to our needs some research/skill icon of 🕮 and the get some real life instruction and do lots of research icon of 🏳. A few things have even earned a 🏳🏳 designation, because they are potentially life threatening or otherwise very dangerous.

How to Use this Checklist

You may want to hold off on doing this checklist until you're a bit more comfortable with BDSM in general. Or you may find it interesting to do the checklist right away, when you're first exploring, so that you can come back to it in a year or so and see what's changed. I know there have been many things that I thought were out of the question when I was new that are now some of my favourite things. The choice is yours!

You may find it easiest to photocopy this list or download it from my website at www.MsMorganThorne.com if you prefer to do it online or print it out yourself. Of course, you're more than welcome to fill out this one right here in the book if you want to keep things all in one place.

Both or all partners should fill out this checklist, to gauge interest in activities and so that they are aware of what the other(s) are interested in. If you have multiple partners, each pairing should fill out a checklist, as what you are willing to explore with one partner may be different than what you are willing to explore with another.

Make sure you indicate your experience, if any, with each activity. Again, this is the beginning of a conversation, not the whole thing. Don't be afraid to ask a person how they learned, whether they were a top or bottom for that activity, etc.

If an activity does not apply to you for whatever reason, simply ignore it or write in **N/A**.
Use a **T** or **B** to indicate that you would be interested in topping or bottoming for an activity. If you're interested in doing both, simply write both letters in.

Rating scale for the checklist. Remember, if you haven't tried an activity, indicate your interest level in that activity. If you plan on having others involved directly in your play, indicate with an * which activities you would want to keep between you and your primary partner or the person you are filling this checklist out with.

- **NO** is a hard limit, something you are not interested in doing under any circumstances.
- **0** (zero) is a soft limit, something you aren't interested in doing, but may consider under specific circumstances and with specific negotiation.
- 1 (one) is something you aren't really interested in doing but will oblige if it's requested occasionally.
- **2** (two) is something that you're okay with doing but you don't really enjoy. You will do it if asked, to please your partner, or as a special reward.
- **3** (three) is something that you neither like nor dislike. You're up for it if your partner wants to, but it's not something you would miss if it didn't happen.
- **4** (four) is something you enjoy doing and wouldn't mind doing often.
- **5** (five) is something you really want to do, something you would like to do as often as possible.
- **?** is something you don't understand or are truly unsure about.

There are blank spots at the end of each checklist. If there is something that fits this category that I haven't included, write it in! I've also done my best to keep the lists somewhat short, which means I've left out some of the more extreme activities. If you are interested in more extreme play, make sure you get educated on how to do it safely, including attending workshops and reading all you can on the subject.

Name: Date:

Taboo & Edge Play Activity	Experience Y/N	Rating NO, 1-5, ?	Top or Bottom
Age Play (Sexual) 🕮			
Animal Role Play (Sexual) 🕮			
Asphyxiation ⚐⚐			
Ball Busting 🕮			
Bare-backing 🕮			
Blackmail Fantasy ⚐			
Blood Play ⚐⚐			
Branding ⚐			
Breath Control ⚐			
Breeding Fantasy			
Castration Fantasy 🕮			
Catheters ⚐⚐			
CBT (Cock & Ball Torture) 🕮			
Choking ⚐⚐			

Taboo & Edge Play Activity	Experience Y/N	Rating NO, 1-5, ?	Top or Bottom
Conditioning (Manipulation) 🏳			
Corporal "Punishment" 🕮 🏳			
Cunt Busting 🕮			
Enemas (Cleansing) 🕮			
Enemas (Pleasure) 🕮			
Enemas (Punishment) 🕮			
Enemas (Retention) 🕮			
Fear Play 🕮			
Fire Play 🕮 🏳			
Flesh Hook Suspension 🏳🏳			
Full Body Beatings 🕮 🏳			
Gas Masks (Air Restriction) 🕮			
Genitorture 🕮			
Gun Play 🕮 🏳			
Golden Showers 🕮			
Gun Play 🏳			
Hypnosis 🕮 🏳			

Taboo & Edge Play Activity	Experience Y/N	Rating NO, 1-5, ?	Top or Bottom
Inflation/Injections (Saline) ⚐⚐			
Interrogations 🕮⚐			
Knife Play 🕮			
Mind Fucks 🕮			
Needle Play ⚐			
Pursuit & Capture (Public) 🕮 ⚐			
Pursuit & Capture (Kink Camping or Similar) 🕮 ⚐			
Play Piercing ⚐			
Pussy Torture 🕮			
Ravishment Play (Rape Play) 🕮 ⚐			
Resistance Play 🕮 ⚐			
Rough Body Play (Closed Fists) 🕮 ⚐			
Rough Body Play (Kicking) 🕮 ⚐			
Scat ⚐			
Sleep Deprivation 🕮			
Stress Positions 🕮 ⚐			
Take Down Play 🕮 ⚐			

Taboo & Edge Play Activity	Experience Y/N	Rating NO, 1-5, ?	Top or Bottom
Tasers/Stun Guns 🕮 ⚐			
Urethral Sounding ⚐			
Urine Consumption 🕮			
Waterboarding ⚐			

40 EXPLORING TABOO & EDGE PLAY: SAFETY

I won't go into a lot of detail on many of these activities. So many of them require serious education before attempting. Where it is reasonable to do so I will provide practical safety advice. This is in no way an alternative to getting properly educated on the subject. Don't try this at home! (unless you've taken a few classes and know what you're doing).

We will start with the taboo activities and safety concerns with those. These are activities that are less dangerous and are simply taboo in nature.

Taboo Safety

Ballbusting is part of the umbrella kink of cock and ball torture. There are numerous dangers associated with these kinks, including infertility and damage to the testicles. Obviously, if you apply a hard enough impact to a testicle, it can rupture. Twisting the scrotum can result in a torsion, which can lead to testicle death in a matter of hours.

Damage to the erectile tissues of the penis, through impact or puncture, can cause erectile dysfunction. Damage to the urethra can cause strictures which can interfere with sexual enjoyment and urination. Banding, a semi-popular kink among castration fetishists, can lead to the loss of the scrotum, penis and can result in gangrene. Banding should never be practised, even temporarily.

CBT can be done safely. If you would like to try, start with very light flicks or taps. You don't need a lot of force to generate a reaction. Very gentle squeezing is fine as well. Anything beyond that should be learned through a workshop.

Cunt busting is the female equivalent of ball busting. There are fewer structures to damage on a vulva because most of the important organs are inside the body. The heavy impact can cause bad bruising and severe pain. Like CBT, start with light slaps and flicks, anything else, take a class.

Barebacking is sex without condoms. With a trusted partner, this is not a high-risk activity. With strangers (as the fetish usually goes), it has high risks of STIs and for some, pregnancy. This is something that you may want to fantasize about, but the reality can leave you open to a host of health issues. Breeding fantasies also have similar risks, including pregnancy (which is the fantasy).

Similarly, blackmail fantasies (exactly what it sounds like) can be fun with a trustworthy partner. With a stranger, it can quickly go from fantasy to actual blackmail. Make sure you negotiate and have trust in the person you give personal information to. You may want to consider a professional dominant in this case, as they have a reputation to protect.

Corporal punishments can range from regular BDSM play to extreme. Make sure that you and your partner are on the same page about what the words mean. You wouldn't want to go in expecting mid-level play where a safeword will be headed when your partner thinks you want extreme pain with safe words ignored.

Enemas are taboo for some because of what gets expelled. For most enema play, the waste is expelled in the toilet and is not part of play. The point is the discomfort, painful cramps and feelings of fullness of the enemas themselves. There is also an element of humiliation play involved too. Enemas are fairly easy to administer but if you want to experiment with different recipes, it's best to do some research. Never add alcohol or drugs to an enema. The body absorbs it much quicker and several people have died that way. You may be able to get away with it a few times, but your luck will run out eventually.

Gas masks used for air restriction and holding your hand over a person's mouth and nose are the safer ways of doing breath play. They are far from safe, anytime you restrict a person's breathing you run the risk of brain damage or death. There are simply safer ways to do it because as soon as you remove your hand (or allow air flow back into the mask), breathing is restored. It is very dangerous to deprive a person of air long enough that they lose consciousness. It can cause brain damage.

Golden showers are probably one of the safer things on this list, but many are put off by the taboo nature of drinking or being covered in urine. If you are consuming urine, make sure the donor is healthy and not on medications which are excreted in urine. If you are getting pissed on without consumption, make sure you don't have any open cuts or wounds that could get infected.

Knife play should not break the skin, it should be a mind fuck or fear play. Most knives are not able to be sterilized appropriately (and I mean actually sterile, not sanitized, not disinfected, not just clean). Anything which is being used to break skin must be sterile and aseptic technique should be observed.

Anytime you're doing public resistance play, you run the risk of someone calling the police. If you want to engage in these sorts of activities, there are numerous kink camping events, across North America, Europe and Australia (and probably in other parts of the world too) that you can attend. They often have space set aside for these sorts of scenes.

Edge Play Safety

Any type of breath play or asphyxiation that involves the throat, blood chokes and similar activities are incredibly dangerous. You can mitigate some of the danger by taking martial arts that teach a blood choke technique, but it is still dangerous. I will not engage in these types of activities, and neither will most health care professionals I know. The risks of brain damage and death are too high.

Catheters and sounding should only be done by people who are trained to do so. Aseptic technique needs to be used and instruments need to be sterile. Even then, both activities leave one vulnerable to infections. Catheters are more dangerous than sounding because of how deep into the body they go. Poor catheter technique can result in urinary incontinence, which may become permanent. Sounding on vulvae is more dangerous than penises because of the much shorter urethra. There is a much higher infection risk.

When done properly, fire play is not that dangerous. You do need to get in-person instruction to learn the appropriate techniques and safety precautions. Choice of fuel will also have an effect on safety.

Flesh hook suspension has all the danger of play piercing doubled because of how deep the piercings are, added to the dangers of rope suspension and bonus risks of skin tearing. Basically, these should never be attempted by untrained persons - and half the people I've seen who claim to be trained (in the BDSM community) are deluding themselves. This is an activity best left up to a reputable suspension team based in the body modification industry.

Play piercings and needle play must be done observing aseptic techniques. Single use, disposable, sterile needles are the only acceptable sharp for this activity. Safety pins, hat pins, etc are made from low-quality metals and cannot be sterilized (again, real sterilization, in an autoclave). Needles should never be driven directly into the body.

Rough body play that involves kicking or closed fists should only be done by those who have appropriate martial arts training. The potential to cause damage to the bottom is very high with these activities.

There are a few things on this list, such as gunplay, that I think are far too dangerous to do at all. Many of the people into that particular kink feel that the precautions needed to make it safer take all the "fun" away. I don't believe that loaded guns and kink should be combined.

So there you have it. A big long list of scary shit. I don't mean to be a downer, but these sorts of play are dangerous. They can be done in ways that make them safer (most of the time), but that takes knowledge and skill. If you don't have both of those, wait to try these things until you do.

41 EXPLORING TABOO & EDGE PLAY: EDUCATIONAL RESOURCES FOR ADVANCED PLAY

So you want to learn advanced play, do you? Whether it's needle play, rope suspension, or single tail whips, the answer is the same: take classes.

Your local community will have a lot of classes on various BDSM techniques. If you don't have a community where you live, check out the nearest big city. Most cities have a BDSM scene and kinksters love workshops.

Most workshops are put on by local people who are accomplished in a particular skill. Sometimes you're able to find travelling instructors who earn a living giving classes on various subjects. Kink conventions are also a fantastic place to learn, as instructors from all over the world travel to these.

Books are a good source of information but are no substitute for the real thing. Be careful, I have seen lots of books trying to cash in on the 50 Shades phenomena that are poorly written by people who don't seem to actually do kink. I remember reading one that talked about mummification (the practice of using strict bondage to wrap a person up, usually with plastic wrap or tape) using linen bandages - as in Egyptian mummy.

If you're going to buy books, check them out first and make sure that they are reputable.

There are also a number of online resources that you can access, for free or for a fee. I would start on the free sites before paying for videos that you are unsure of the quality. I shouldn't have to say it, but porn is not instructional. I've worked in the industry briefly and found that many of the actors aren't even kinky, never mind skilled.

In the back of this book, I will include links to the various other educational resources I produce, including books, videos, articles and in-person classes.

I mentioned in the bondage section two worldwide groups for learning shibari style rope bondage. Hitchin' Bitches have groups all over the world in many major cities that are dedicated to women and femme rope tops. People of all genders are welcome to participate as bottoms, but only women and femmes are allowed to tie.

Rope bite is another well known international group. They are open to everyone who wants to learn rope and have a range of instruction from beginner to more advanced. They usually have open practice times as well.

Many communities host travelling rope instructors who share their knowledge. If you have an interest in a certain person's style, you may be able to take a class or two when they're in town.

Connecting to your local community is the way to access many of these resources. Munches, gatherings of kinky people in pubs or coffee shops, are a basic meet and greet tool. They are the gateway to the rest of the community.

You can find what local resources are available to you by joining Fetlife.com, a free social networking site for kinky people. I'm not crazy about the site, but it is the largest of its kind and free is always a nice price.

42 CREATING AMAZING SCENES

This is it, you've tried out many of the most popular types of play in the BDSM realm. You have a good idea of what you like and what is not so hot. You've learned some very important communication skills, how to negotiate, and how to obtain consent in the world of kink. You're off to a great start.

The last thing you will need to know is how to combine all of those elements to create an amazing scene. There are a lot of elements that contribute to an amazing scene, so let's take a look at them now.

Setting the Mood

Setting the mood for kinky play isn't that much different than setting the mood for a romantic vanilla night. Think of the things you would want for that and you're well on your way to a great kink scene.

Music can play an important role in your scene. Not only does it provide a backdrop to the scene, it can cover or muffle noises that you don't want nosy neighbours to hear. It can help set the mood of the scene. A slow, ominous soundtrack can set a sombre mood for funishment play, while a light, an upbeat song can be a lot of fun for a tickle scene.

I find that I love listening to certain types of music for certain types of play. Faster songs are great for canning, you can strike with the beat. Flogging is better with something a little bit slower, but heavier. Each strike can land in time with the music and create a really cool effect. I've also been known to dance around to the music while playing, using it to inspire me to wonderful acts of sadism.

If you're into role play, costumes can be a lot of fun. You can even dress up your bedroom or wherever it is your scene is taking place. You don't need anything too fancy, just an accent piece here or there can help create a new backdrop for your scene.

Getting dressed up for scenes, even when you're playing at home, makes them feel a bit more special. I love my fetish clothing and I don't get enough of an excuse to wear it lately. I might as well get all dolled up for the home dungeon. It also helps with some types of play. If I want to do a boot worship scene, black leather stiletto boots look a bit strange paired with whatever yoga pants I was wearing that day. A black wet look dress and a corset can really bring the whole thing together.

I love going to the November 1st sales after Halloween. You can pick up all sorts of cool costume and decor accents for half the price of the day before. Use these sales to find cute pieces that will help turn your bedroom from the suburbs to dungeon chic.

Setting the Scene

Depending on the type of scene you're doing, you may want to add a little drama to the beginning. If you're doing a funishment scene, having your "prisoner" locked up on a chair facing the wall while you change can add to the fun. A naughty student can be set to writing lines before the teacher arrives.

Having the bottom carefully lay out your implements before a scene can get them in a good headspace. It can create tension or anticipation. You may be kind and allow them to add one item from the toy stash that they would enjoy. If you're even nicer, you could allow them to take away one item and replace it with something different.

Sometimes you will want to do that sort of work yourself. I love having my bottom tied up and watching while I slowly pull out one toy after another. I like to take a long look at each one, letting them use their imagination to anticipate what's about to happen. Sometimes if I'm feeling mean, I will throw in something scary that I don't intend to use, like a giant rubber fist or a meat hook. When you have a reputation as a sadist, these little mind fucks are too easy.

Of course, you may just want to be left alone to lay out your toys and go over your plan for the scene in your head. Some people find that this is a time for them to focus and get into the right headspace for play.

Don't rush this part, however you want to do it. This is your time to make sure you have everything you need (and maybe a few things you don't). If there is something you want to surprise (in a consensual way, more on that in a minute) your bottom with, send them for a glass of water or ice so you can hide the surprise without them seeing.

The Element of Surprise

Whenever I teach classes on BDSM basics or negotiation/consent, people always have the same argument against it. They want to surprise their partner. Now, I have no idea why you would want to surprise someone with a sexual or physical act without confirming first that they're into it, but I've been kinky for a very long time and we just don't do that.

If you want to surprise your bottom with an activity in a scene, have them consent to a list of activities. Include some things you don't plan on doing, some things you want to do and hide the surprise in the middle. They will know that you won't be doing everything on the list, but they won't know which activities you will choose to use.

The other way is to fill out a master checklist, with all sorts of activities on it (page). Ask if they're okay giving blanket consent to things they've indicated are 4/5 or better. Or fill out a checklist specifically for "pre-consent" so that you have a list of the things you can surprise them with.

In kink, we need to make sure our partners are consenting to the things we do. They are assault if they aren't consenting. These are things that could land us in jail. Aside from that, who wants to harm or violate their partner anyway? These are people we are supposed to care about.

We've come up with some creative ways to get that consent and still be able to surprise our partners. For us, the surprise is not in the what, but more the when.

The Structure of a Scene

Scenes will generally follow the same pattern, in the same way that a story follows a basic structure or a song does. We start with a warm-up, build to an apex, then the ending.

We already covered the warm-up at the beginning of the book. Take your time with it, there's no need to rush. You're looking for a few things before you move on to the next step in play. If you're doing impact play, you want to see the skin pink and warm to the touch. It should almost radiate heat. Your partner should also be relaxed and into the scene.

This can look a number of different ways. They may be very mellow and be moaning. They could be giddy and giggly. They may be energetic and excited. Maybe they're being a bit bratty and bantering with you. Part of it will depend on the mood you've set and the activities you've chosen to do. Part of it will depend on the personality of the bottom and your relationship.

Once you're happy with your warm up, you want to start building towards the apex. This will be the most intense the play gets during the scene. It's also where you should pull out the special toys. Depending on what you have planned, you want to save the best for the apex.

What you should be focusing on right now is building sensation, building intensity. No matter what type of play you're doing, you should be able to slowly turn up the dial. This should be the bulk of your scene. Take your time and enjoy.

When the time is right, hit the apex of play. This is where you want to use the meanest implements, the best vibrator, the nastiest insults, or the sensuous toys. If you're planning a surprise, this is the time.

Think of it like sex, you've spent all this time building up to an orgasm, so make it a good one.

This will probably be the shortest part of your scene but the most intense. The warm-up, the slow build, have all lead to this point where the senses are almost overloaded. It can be helpful to let the bottom know that this is as intense as it gets. You may want them to count hard strikes with the cane, beg for mercy while you tickle them, or tell them it's almost over as you place pressure on the ties binding them.

What happens next can vary, depending on the scene and the bottom.

Some bottoms like to end on a high note. Again, it's like an orgasm, once it happens, they just want to roll over and go to sleep. Talk to your bottom beforehand and find out what they prefer. If they are unsure, you can play it by ear, seeing how they react if you stop the scene at the end of the heavy cane strikes (or whatever your apex was).

Sometimes it's better to do a cooldown, pretty much the opposite of a warm up. You slowly go lighter and lighter, easing your bottom closer to the end of the scene. This way of ending a scene will feel less abrupt and it's a good way to transition into aftercare. Some scenes have it built in. A rope bondage scene will have a slow come down as you untie. You can make this very connective and sensual if you choose.

Some will not like a gentle come down after the scene. They wanted the hard ending. Others can feel abandoned with a hard ending, it's too abrupt for them. You will have to figure out what works best for your bottom and play style.

Aftercare

Once the scene is over, it's time to start your aftercare, if you want to engage in it. If you're playing in a public dungeon, it's expected that you will clean up the play station before moving to the aftercare area. Don't do your aftercare in the play area and don't leave things a mess to clean up after you're done your aftercare.

If you're playing at home, you can clean up right away if you want or leave it for a while. I find that I prefer to clean up right away, while I still have the buzz from the scene, rather than wait and find I'm exhausted.

Combining Elements

Now that you have a basic idea of how a scene should progress - low and slow, building up to a high point, then coming back down, a bit quicker than you built things up. You can now add together different elements from the various areas we've experimented with. Combine bondage, impact, sensation and humiliation. Or power exchange, role play and pain play. Whatever combination works for you.

Don't get too carried away though. You still want to keep the number of activities low. I will usually stick to the 3-5 rule for an hour of play. It gives me time to explore each element of the scene and I don't feel rushed or overwhelmed. If you're doing activities like impact, you can use a few implements and call it one thing. It doesn't take much to switch between a paddle, cane and crop.

Reread the list of first-timer mistakes (page 63) to ensure that you don't get too carried away with trying new combinations and too many activities.

You will quickly learn which activities work well together for your own personal playstyle. As I warned at the beginning of the book, don't try to mix too many activities that require a lot of set up. Ideally, you want to keep it to one per scene, with the rest of the activities being things you can do quickly and easily.

Creativity

You will quickly learn that the most important tool in your BDSM arsenal is creativity. Your imagination will allow you to create the most amazing scenes if you let it. Don't be afraid to think big and take some chances at feeling silly. If you have a great scene idea, suggest it. If you can do it in a safe manner, someone is likely to take you up on your offer (if you play with multiple people). The most popular kinksters are the ones who are willing to put themselves out there and risk feeling silly.

In my local community, there is a dominant who is well known for his "Chicken Florentine". This gruff looking dominant will be flogging a bottom hard then pull out two rubber chickens from his toy bag. Florentine is a flogging style which uses two floggers simultaneously. For Chicken Florentine, replace the floggers with rubber chickens. It always gets a laugh out of anyone watching. The bottoms range from humiliated to amazed a rubber chicken can hurt that much.

If you can be creative and get into your scenes, whether it's a role play or something else entirely, you will have fun. Use your imagination, your sense of humour, and your perverted mind to take your bottom on a wonderful journey into your twisted mind. Take your bottoms suggestions on board as well. Good bottoms have a way of throwing themselves under the bus by suggesting the most painful, most humiliating, most wonderfully awful scenes.

You've had a chance to explore some of the most popular aspects of BDSM. You've learned the importance of consent and built valuable experiences negotiating simple scenes. Hopefully, you've been able to communicate with your partner(s) in an honest and thoughtful manner, so that you can explore in a mutually satisfying way. You're well on your way to becoming the kinky person you always wanted to be.

Now put the book down, it’s time to go and explore BDSM!

Glossary

- **24/7** - Engaging in D/s roles at all times.
- **Abuse** - Actions done without consent. Can be physical or emotional. Manipulating a person so they do what you want.
- **Age Play** - Play where a person assumes a different age, taking on mannerisms of that age group
- **Aftercare** - Wind down time that happens after a play scene. Can involve anything the parties involved need. Common aftercare consists of cuddling, a snack, a cup of tea/glass of wine, talking, or anything else that works for those involved.
- **BDSM** - Bondage, Discipline/Domination, Sadism/Submission, Masochism. Catch-all term for kinky sex and play, power exchange relationships and all things not "vanilla"
- **Bedroom-Only** - BDSM or D/s activities are only engaged in during sexual intimacy or in the bedroom.
- **Bondage** - Restraining a person. May involve rope, handcuffs, leather cuffs or straps, bondage tape, pallet or plastic wrap, vacuum beds, or any other device that restricts movement.
    - Also **Mental Bondage** - Commanding a person not move or restricting their movements by giving an order.
- **Bottom** - The person receiving the sensations or actions
- **Bottom Space** - See "Subspace"
- **Consent** - Giving agreement to participate in an activity, after weighing the risks vs rewards without pressure or coercion.
    - Also **Implied Consent** - The assumption of permission due to past consent or relationship expectations.
    - Also **Blanket Consent** - Permission granted for an activity at any time in the future or permission for a wide range of activities that can be done at any time.

    - Also **Informed Consent** - Understanding the realistic and potential risks associated with an activity and agreeing to participate in it without pressure or coercion.
    - Also **Enthusiastic Consent** - Gleefully agreeing to participate in an activity, understanding the potential risks and without pressure or coercion.
    - Also **Affirmative Consent or Expressed Consent** - The idea that only "yes" means "yes" and that anything else means "no".
- **Consensual Non-Consent (CNC)** - A relationship style where one person agrees to obey the other at all times. If they don't, the Dominant person can simply do what they like (within negotiated boundaries), relying on prior, blanket consent. See also: Resistance Play
- **D/s** - Dominant/submissive. A power exchange relationship where one partner consensually gives up power or authority to another in specific parts of life or overall.
- **Discipline** - Punishment for breaking agreed upon rules.
- **Dominant** - The person who assumes power or authority in a power exchange relationship.
    - A gender neutral term for a Dominant person; can be shortened to **Dom**
    - Also **Domme** - A faux french word to denote a Dominant who is a woman.
- **Dominatrix** - A professional Dominant woman.
- **Dom Space** - See "Top Space"
- **Dungeon** Monitor - A volunteer who is responsible for enforcing the house rules at a play party, ensures safety of players. Often shortened to DM
- **Edge Play** - Play which is generally considered to be more dangerous (needle play, knife play, fire play, etc)
- **Fetish** - Sexual arousal caused by an object or part of the body which is not typically considered to be sexual, ie. foot fetish
    - Sometimes misused to indicate any type of interest in kinky activities.
- **Fetishist** - A person with one or more sexual fetishes.
- **Funishment** - Role-played punishments. Giving a punishment because all parties involved erotocise punishment, not because rules or agreements were broken.
- **Genitorture** - Play that involves causing pain to the genitals
- **Green** - A less used safe word to indicate that everything is great. Used as part of a check-in during play "What colour are you?" "Green!" Part of the stoplight safe word system.
- **Hedonist** - A person who seeks pleasure for pleasure's sake. A person to whom the pursuit of pleasure is the most important part of life. It is part philosophy and part action.
- **Humiliation** - A form of emotional sadism or masochism that often involves name calling, embarrassing situations, or public shaming.

    - Also **Degradation** - A more extreme form of humiliation which removes the humanity of the person being degraded. Can include the above elements of humiliation as well.
    - Also **Objectification** - Reducing a person to an object and using them as such. Popular themes include human furniture, sex toy, and sushi platter
- **Kink** - Activities pertaining to BDSM or fetishes.
- **Kinkster** - A person who engages in kink or BDSM
- **Land-mine** - Typically, a trigger that the person wasn't aware of. Can be found during certain types of play, humiliation play is most common.
- **Limits** - Things you are uninterested in doing within a BDSM context. Can be anything you can think of from activities to using specific words.
    - Also **Hard Limit** - A thing you will not do under any circumstances, no way, no how.
    - Also **Soft Limit** - A thing you do not enjoy doing, but may consider doing with the right person and/or under the right circumstances.
- **Mistress** - A term that some women who are Dominant prefer to be called.
    - Sometimes can denote a Professional Dominant woman.
- **Masochism** - Getting pleasure through consensually applied pain.
- **Master** - A gender neutral term that some Dominant people prefer to be called.
    - A person who owns a consensual slave or property.
    - A person who has achieved a high level of skill in a particular area.
    - A person who has earned their title in the Leather tradition of BDSM.
- **Mummification** - Wrapping a person so they can not move at all. Usually involves plastic or pallet wrap, duct tape, and other materials that can be wrapped tightly around the body. Vacuum beds, made from latex, are also popular among people who enjoy mummification.
- **Negotiation** - Discussing what each person would like to get out of a BDSM scene or relationship and coming to an agreement about what actions will take place or how the relationship will be structured.
    - An essential skill to learn in BDSM, how one obtains consent to engage in kinky activities or relationships.
- **Power Exchange Relationship** - An arrangement or relationship where one partner consensually gives up authority over parts or all of their life to the other partner.
- **Punishment** - Genuine reprimand, often in physical form, for breaking agreed upon rules.
- **Red** - One of the universal safe words. Generally means stop all play, the scene is over OR check in and find out what's wrong, go from there. Part of the stoplight safe word system.
- **Resistance Play** - Play scenes where one party is free to yell or say "no", "stop", without actually meaning it. Common forms of resistance play can include rape/ravishment play, kidnap scenes, and other "distress" style scenes. It is always

wise to have a safe word to indicate problems or a withdrawal of consent, since "no" will be ignored. Should not be confused with Consensual Non-Consent.

- **Role Play** - Taking on the persona of another person or a character. Can be general (teacher and student) or fictional characters.
- **Sadism** - Getting pleasure through causing consensual pain to another
- **Sadomasochist** - A person who enjoys both causing and receiving consensual pain.
- **Safe Word or Signal** - A way to indicate that something has gone wrong during a scene.
    - A way to signal that you have withdrawn consent for the activities you are engaged in.
    - Safe word refers to a code word that can be spoken to really mean "no, stop" during a struggle or resistance scene.
    - Safe signal refers to an object that can be dropped or shaken to make noise, a hand signal, a tap, etc, that indicates a problem when a person is bound or gagged in such a way that verbal communication is difficult or impossible.
    - Safe words and signals are negotiated in advance, all parties must agree on what they are and what they mean.
- **Shibari** - Japanese rope bondage that creates beautiful and elaborate ties, often within certain pre-determined forms (box tie, shrimp tie, etc).
    - Used by some to describe rope bondage as art or performance.
    - Also **Kinbaku** - Often interchangeable with Shibari.
        - Used by some to describe rope bondage that is intricate, beautiful, connective and sexually or sensually arousing.
- **Slave** - A person who gives up all authority to another in a power exchange relationship.
    - A person who is consensually owned property
    - A hot name to call your partner during a Master/Mistress & slave roleplay session.
- **Submissive** - The person who gives up power or authority in a power exchange relationship.
    - A gender neutral title for a person who identifies as submissive; can be shortened to **sub**.
- **Subspace (Bottom Space)** - A somewhat controversial state of mind where the submissive/bottom experiences intense feelings. Often described as 'floaty' or a feeling of being high, it is thought to be caused by the endorphin rush associated with intense play. Others argue that it is not related to physical sensation, and say they can achieve it by words alone.
  Not everyone is able to achieve subspace or even wants to. It should not be expected to happen in every play scene. Rather it is an occasional state that some find very enjoyable.
  It should be noted that subspace is considered to be an altered state of mind, much

like imbibing alcohol. Scenes should not be re-negotiated when a person is in this state.

- **Top Space (Dom Space)** - A less common term used to describe a flow state that many Dominants or Tops achieve while playing. This is similar to the flow state felt by artists or athletes who are in "the zone".
- **Total Power Exchange** - The dominant partner is in charge of all aspects of the relationship and the submissive's life.
- **Vanilla** - A person who is not into kink or BDSM.
    - An activity which is not considered to be kinky
    - Sometimes used as a slur, but generally value neutral.
- **What It Is We Do** - A way to talk about kink, BDSM. An umbrella term that encompasses the different ways people do BDSM or kink.
- **Yellow** - A somewhat lesser used universal safe word to indicate that a person is close to their limit and in need of less intensity. Can also mean that the person can not tolerate any further use of the current implement or that they need the Top/Dom to slow down or ease up. Part of the stoplight safe word system.

ABOUT MORGAN THORNE

Morgan Thorne has been practising BDSM all her adult life. She got an introduction to kink through the Queer community in the early 1990's and knew she had found 'her people'. Morgan has also spent nearly a decade working as a Professional Dominant, which has allowed her to expand her skills as both a Top and a Dominant. Morgan has been offering workshops, lectures and BDSM training for a number of years as well. She has a successful Youtube channel where she educates about D/s relationships, BDSM basics and various kinky skills.

Morgan identifies as both a Sadist and a Dominant. She enjoys playing with a variety of people of all orientations/genders/identities. BDSM is an integral part of her personal, romantic relationships. Morgan is both asexual and pan-romantic.

Prior to her work as a Professional Dominant, Morgan worked in health care. This has allowed her to gain a more thorough understanding of health and safety concerns in kink. She retired due to an injury that lead to chronic pain and disability. It also lead to her interest in medical play, a way to continue to use the skills she learned in health care and to find comfort in the loss of a much-loved career.

Morgan has been active in various forms of activism, including LGBTQIA rights and sex worker rights. She is a strong advocate for equality and the human rights of all people.

CONNECT WITH MORGAN

Keep up to date on my website: www.MsMorganThorne.com

Subscribe to my Youtube channel
for FREE BDSM instructional videos: www.Youtube.com/MorganThorneBDSM

Follow me on Instagram: www.Instagram.com/MsMorganThorne

Follow me on Twitter: www.Twitter.com/Nymphetamean

Friend me on Fetlife: MorganThorne

Join me on Facebook: www.Facebook.com/MsMorganThorne

OTHER TITLES BY MORGAN THORNE

A Guide to Classic Discipline

In her debut book, Morgan Thorne writes about the art and practice of Classic Discipline, also known as English Discipline.

We begin with a quick lesson on the history of classic discipline so that we can use the past as inspiration for our play. Starting with the naval discipline made famous by the British, we continue on to British school discipline, which was (and sometimes still is) used in various parts of the world to keep students in line. We finish up with ritual and religious discipline, a taboo subject that many find erotic.

Getting into the practical side of BDSM practice begins with exploring different types of consent, negotiation and when a 'safe word' may be needed. The differences between punishments and 'funishments' are examined, with instructions and advice for engaging in both. Morgan is well known for her emphasis on safety and goes into thorough detail on how to stay safe, both in body and mind.

It is then time to learn how to use a variety of implements, including different techniques, where on the body to use them, and how to care for the implement. The book covers canes, floggers, straps, paddles, switches, birches and many other implements that fall into the category of classic discipline.

This book covers what you need to know to create your own kinky discipline scenes, including how to structure your scene for different styles of play. Whether it's a punishment cold caning or a more sensual flogging scene with a schoolyard twist, a Guide to Classic Discipline will provide you with what you need to know.

Available on Amazon in both print and e-book format.

COMING IN 2018

MEDICAL ASEPTIC TECHNIQUE FOR BDSM

I have two big passions in my life; all things medical and all things BDSM. I have been lucky enough to have the opportunity to pursue both over the course of my life and now I enjoy combining the two.

Unfortunately for me, my pursuit of the medical field ended early when I suffered a life changing and disabling injury during the course of my workday.

I decided to enter the world of professional domination.

As I was exploring this new vocation, I quickly learned that 'medical play' was quite popular. I also found that as I accepted the loss of my career, I began to enjoy medical play myself. Before, it was work. Now it became an outlet for that passion, which I could share with others in a non-traditional way. I embraced medical play and strove to learn as much as I could, applying my formal training to this new avenue of expression.

I discovered that many kinksters either didn't know or didn't care about the technical side of things. They didn't understand why sterility was important (essential) in some circumstances, or how to avoid cross-contamination.

When I started teaching different medical play techniques, people flocked to my classes to learn. There are bottoms out there who will not play with someone unless they have attended my classes and follow appropriate medical aseptic technique.

It's not as if I have been teaching anything revolutionary. This is standard practice for any medical professional.

As I grow as a BDSM educator, I have more and more people asking to learn these techniques. I decided to write this book for those people, so that they can gain what I consider to be essential knowledge for anyone engaging in many forms of medical play, tailored for BDSM practice. This book is written using plain language where possible and gives definitions or thorough explanations of any technical terms that are used. I want to share my passion for this style of kink, as well as do what I can to help keep people safe. It is the perfect combination of my two passions.

I hope that you find this information useful, easy to understand and implement in your scenes. As kinksters, I believe that we should always strive to do things better and in a safer manner, so that our partners and friends take on less risk in playing with us.

Made in United States
North Haven, CT
11 March 2022

17053758R00172